LIPPINCOTT WILLIAMS & WILKINS'

Certification Preparation
for Dental Assisting

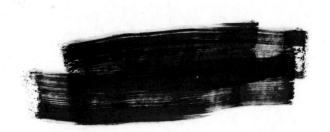

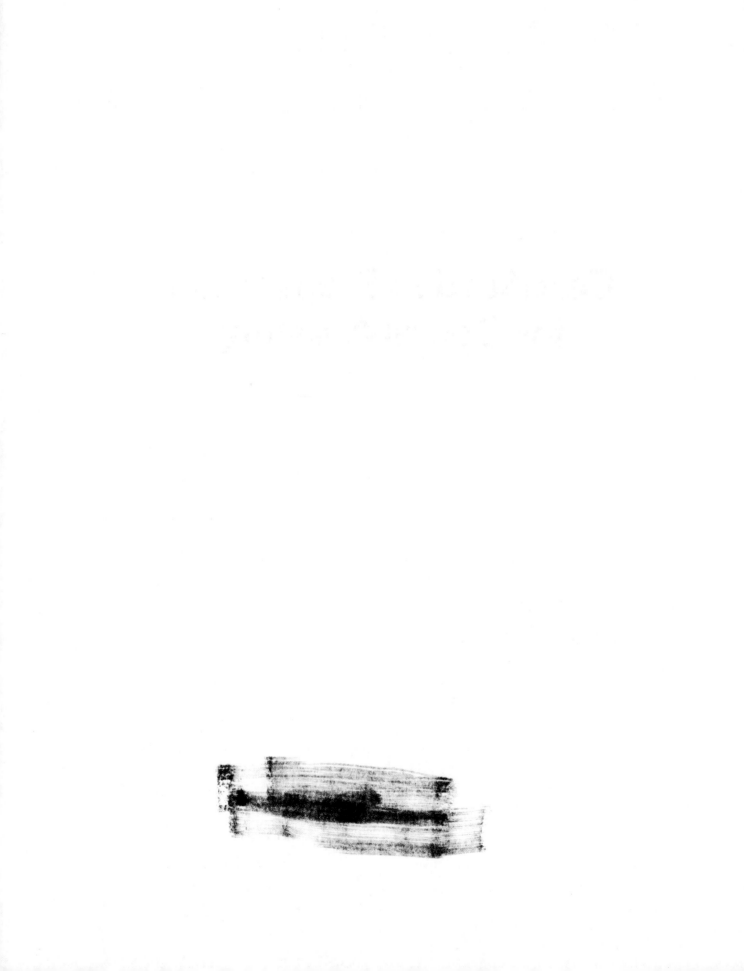

LIPPINCOTT WILLIAMS & WILKINS'

Certification Preparation for Dental Assisting

Wolters Kluwer | Lippincott Williams & Wilkins
Health

Philadelphia • Baltimore • New York • London
Buenos Aires • Hong Kong • Sydney • Tokyo

Senior Publisher: Julie K. Stegman
Acquisitions Editor: Peter Sabatini
Product Director: Eric Branger
Senior Product Manager: Heather A. Rybacki
Product Manager: Michael Marino
Marketing Manager: Shauna Kelley
Development Editor: Tom Lochhaas
Manufacturing Coordinator: Margie Orzech-Zeranko
Design Coordinator: Steve Druding
Compositor: Absolute Service, Inc.

First Edition

Copyright © 2012 Lippincott Williams & Wilkins, a Wolters Kluwer business

351 West Camden Street   Two Commerce Square
Baltimore, MD 21201   2001 Market Street
                                Philadelphia, PA 19103

Printed in China

9 8 7 6 5 4 3 2 1

Library of Congress Cataloging-in-Publication Data

Cataloging-in-Publication data is available on request.

DISCLAIMER

Care has been taken to confirm the accuracy of the information present and to describe generally accepted practices. However, the authors, editors, and publisher are not responsible for errors or omissions or for any consequences from application of the information in this book and make no warranty, expressed or implied, with respect to the currency, completeness, or accuracy of the contents of the publication. Application of this information in a particular situation remains the professional responsibility of the practitioner; the clinical treatments described and recommended may not be considered absolute and universal recommendations.

The authors, editors, and publisher have exerted every effort to ensure that drug selection and dosage set forth in this text are in accordance with the current recommendations and practice at the time of publication. However, in view of ongoing research, changes in government regulations, and the constant flow of information relating to drug therapy and drug reactions, the reader is urged to check the package insert for each drug for any change in indications and dosage and for added warnings and precautions. This is particularly important when the recommended agent is a new or infrequently employed drug.

Some drugs and medical devices presented in this publication have Food and Drug Administration (FDA) clearance for limited use in restricted research settings. It is the responsibility of the health care provider to ascertain the FDA status of each drug or device planned for use in their clinical practice.

To purchase additional copies of this book, call our customer service department at **(800) 638-3030** or fax orders to **(301) 223-2320**. International customers should call **(301) 223-2300**.

Visit Lippincott Williams & Wilkins on the Internet: **http://www.lww.com.** Lippincott Williams & Wilkins customer service representatives are available from 8:30 am to 6:00 pm, EST.

Contributors and Reviewers

Jessica L. Fisher, CDA, EFDA, CPT, BLS, AASCJ
Director of Dental Assisting
FORTIS College, Indianapolis, Indiana

Teresa A. Macauley, CDA, EFDA, MS
Associate Professor of Health Sciences
Ivy Tech Community College, Anderson, Indiana

Diana L. Olsen, CDA, CDPMA, RDH, EFDA, MS
Coordinator and Adjunct Instructor, EFDA Program
York County Community College, Wells, Maine

Helene A. Pizzuta, CDA, RDA
Dental Program Director
American Institute, Clifton, New Jersey

REVIEWERS

Leora Harty
Medical Careers Institute, Newport News, Virginia

Carole Landes
Everest University, Largo, Florida

Mark Matney
Chattanooga State Community College, Chattanooga, Tennessee

Julie Muhle
Truckee Meadows Community College, Reno, Nevada

Carrie Olewinski
Carrington College, Boise, Idaho

Diana Romero
Delta Tech, Lake Charles, Louisiana

Contents

part I

Preparing for the Dental Assisting National Certification Exam

The Certification Exam

Why get DANB certified? Why go through the hassle, the added time, and the pressure of taking a national board exam to prove your credentials? The answer is relatively simple. Dentists generally would like their patients to respect and trust them and possibly even recommend them to other potential patients. If that isn't the case, those dentists will soon find their practices dwindling. In order to win patients' trust and respect, it is not enough for only the dentist display a high degree of knowledge and professionalism; the entire dental staff should be held to high expectations as well. A dentist could seek and hire qualified dental assistants based on their word alone ("Sure, I'm qualified!"), but chances are, most dentists will require some documentation as proof that the candidate is, indeed, a qualified professional. To ensure a reputation of excellence for themselves and for their staff, many dentists may require the national certification for employment, even though it may not be a state requirement. Therefore, even if your state does not require taking a credentialing exam such as the DANB, obtaining and maintaining this national credential will speak volumes about your qualifications, professionalism, dedication, and sincerity in being a dental assistant. Frame your certificate and display it proudly where patients can see it! Showing that you are a highly qualified professional will instill patient confidence in your abilities.

As you may already know, the Dental Assisting National Board, Inc. (DANB) is the foremost recognized certification and credentialing agency for dental assistants and is a member of the Institute for Credentialing Excellence (formerly NOCA). Certification by a nationally recognized leader in dental assisting qualifications has many benefits. DANB-certified assistants usually receive higher salaries than their noncredentialed colleagues, and DANB-certification is a requirement for dental assistants to provide expanded functions in many states.

The two areas of certification that are open to eligible candidates are:

- Certified Dental Assistant (CDA)
- Certified Orthodontic Assistant (COA)

Note: This book covers preparation for only the DANB CDA exam.

Computerized Exam

The DANB exam is only administered as a computerized exam. A written version is no longer available. The test is administered year-round at over 200 testing centers across the country. Applications may be turned in at any time, and candidates may schedule their exam online at any time after receiving their test admission notice. The exam must be taken during a 60-day eligibility window. For further information and test center locations, visit the DANB website (www.danb.org).

The Exam Components

The CDA exam consists of three component exams: General Chairside (GC), Radiation Health and Safety (RHS), and Infection Control (ICE). General information about each of these exams—such as the allotted testing time, the total number of questions (items) in each component, and the percentage (%) of exam questions in each topic area—is provided here.

General Chairside (GC) Exam

- 120 multiple-choice items
- 90 minutes (1.5 hours) testing time
- Topics:
  - Collection and recording of clinical data (10%, 12 questions)
  - Chairside dental procedures (45%, 54 questions)
  - Chairside dental materials (preparation, manipulation, application) (11%, 13 questions)
  - Lab materials and procedures (4%, 5 questions)
  - Patient education and oral health management (10%, 12 questions)
  - Prevention and management of emergencies (14%, 17 questions)
  - Office management procedures (6%, 7 questions)

Radiation Health and Safety (RHS) Exam

- 100 multiple-choice items
- 75 minutes (1.25 hours) testing time

- Topics:
  - Exposing and evaluating radiographs (intraoral, extraoral) (37%, 37 questions)
  - Processing films (16%, 16 questions)
  - Mounting/labeling films (11%, 11 questions)
  - Radiation safety, patient (24%, 24 questions)
  - Radiation safety, operator (12%, 12 questions)

Infection Control (ICE) Exam

- 100 multiple-choice items
- 75 minutes (1.25 hours) testing time
- Topics:
  - Patient and dental health care worker education (10%, 10 questions)
  - Prevention of cross-contamination and transmission (20%, 20 questions)
  - Maintaining aseptic conditions (10%, 10 questions)
  - Performing sterilization procedures (15%, 15 questions)
  - Environmental asepsis (15%, 15 questions)
  - Occupational safety (30%, 30 questions)

In total, you will answer 320 multiple-choice items in 4 hours. For each component exam, there are minimum performance standards that you must meet in order to earn the CDA certification. It is to your advantage to know the percentage of questions that will appear for each topic on the exam so that you can schedule your study time accordingly. For example, you should allot more time and energy to studying chairside dental procedures because these questions make up 45% (54 questions) of the GC component exam rather than lab materials and procedures because only 4% (5 questions) of the GC component exam address that topic.

The Exam Questions

The DANB national exam follows strict guidelines. The questions are written in a straightforward style with simple vocabulary; they are not written to trick you into answering incorrectly. Strategies for answering exam questions are provided later in the section, Answering Exam Questions.

The exam is written in a simple multiple-choice format, which asks you to answer in one of two ways:

- Direct-question format: You must answer a direct question by choosing one BEST or MOST CORRECT answer from a choice of possible answers.
- Incomplete-statement format: You much complete an open-ended statement by choosing one BEST or MOST CORRECT word or phrase from a choice of four possible answers.
- Negative format: The DANB exam does not contain many of these types of questions, but it does contain a few. These are questions in which you must find an EXCEPTION or determine which choice is NOT appropriate for the question.

Matching items, true/false items, and questions that could have more than one possible answer, such as "both A and B," "None of the above," or "All of the above," are not used on the DANB exam.

Studying Ahead for the Exam

One of the most important aspects of studying for an exam is not to "study" for the exam at all. Yes, you read that right! But isn't this book designed to help you study for the test? Yes, of course it is. However, many students confuse "studying" with "cramming" for an exam. "Cramming" as much information into your head in a day or two—or even an hour or two—before taking the exam is *not* really "studying." To truly study is to come prepared to each class throughout the academic term, read the material for that day, take notes on the material, and gain a deeper-than-surface-level understanding of the topic. Studying is a wide-ranging commitment. So, to clarify the meaning of the opening sentence: Don't study for the exam, study for the knowledge. Then review for the exam and pass. Studying and reviewing go hand in hand. "Reviewing" for an exam is going back over the material you have already learned and internalized in order to freshen it in your mind.

A great way to begin to truly study is by implementing some long-term studying strategies and methods into your student life.

Set Up Your Study Space

The most important thing you need to know before you get started is what type of environment, or study space, is most conducive to your needs. Ask yourself some very simple questions:

- Where can I be most organized?
- What type of sounds do I like to hear when I'm learning?
- When during the day am I most alert and most receptive to new information?
- How do I best learn?

Some people think the dining room table is a great place to study (and for them it might be), because it may be large and desklike. However, if that means having to put away all study materials at every mealtime or trying to study in the center of a large and/or loud household, it may actually be the least conducive place. Find a space where you can be consistently organized and where your highlighters, notebooks, a computer (if necessary), textbooks, and other study materials can stay and be easily and readily accessible. Your study space should also not be cluttered with other items that could possibly be a distraction, such as phones, pictures, hobbies, magazines, and the like.

Many instructors have argued for studying in a noiseless room. That seems to make a lot of sense—fewer distractions, comfortable, and quiet. However, this may not work for you at all. Utter silence can be deafening and distracting in itself to some people. If you know that you concentrate better when listening to soft music in the background, by all means, do that. (Just be sure that the sound level is truly beneficial to studying, not to dancing and singing along.) By the same token, if you like the sounds of nature, study outside (weather permitting), but go elsewhere if you become distracted by sounds of lawnmowers and heavy traffic. Maybe an indoor room with the window slightly open would serve you better. In the end, you know best what works for you.

Set Up a Study Method

It is important to be aware of how you learn best. If you are an auditory learner—you prefer to hear the information spoken—consider reading your information or text into a recording device and playing back for yourself. This means you can study while driving, jogging, or even while taking the dog for a walk! If you are a visual learner—preferring to see a visual representation of the material—then draw some pictures of the material. If you are not an artist, take photographs. Need to memorize lab materials and proper procedures? Take pictures of them and use those as flashcards. If you learn best by discussing the material to be learned, join or create a study group with other vocal learners. You could also explain the material to an interested friend or relative, or even to your pet. (Don't laugh, it works!) In short, get creative. You know how you learn best. However, if you have any question about it, there are a number of free online sites (such as www.learning-styles-online.com) that will test your learning style and give you results with suggestions for how to make your learning style work for you.

Set Up a Study Schedule

Are you most alert in the morning, afternoon, or evening? This is the time when your mind is most receptive to new and challenging thoughts, so you should schedule your study sessions for those times. If this is not a realistic option because of your work schedule, school, or other obligations, try to get as close as possible to your ideal time or work out a study schedule in which you can study at your best time at least two to three times a week.

Carving out time to study from your other activities is a must, and creating a study schedule will help you stick to a routine and build great study habits. As you create your study schedule, don't forget to include break times of 5 to 10 minutes every 45 minutes or so. Your brain needs downtime to absorb new information, and your body needs a break to relax and de-stress from studying.

Make sure that you don't schedule your study time immediately after a heavy meal or after a hectic or stressful time of day. What you put into your body and what type of stress you place on your body directly affect how efficiently your mind works, how readily you absorb information, and how accurately you retain and recall material. Eating right, exercising, getting enough sleep, and taking frequent relaxation breaks will help the knowledge be absorbed.

The Process of Studying

When you have considered all these options, then you are ready to get down to the business of studying. Obviously, you should study your dental assisting textbook. Focus your reading by asking questions and answering those questions while you read. Think:

- When will I most likely need to use this fact, procedure, or idea?
- How would this be phrased as an exam question?
- What is the next step in this procedure? How does it relate to the step before?
- Does this make sense?

If it helps you, write down the questions (and answers). If you come across a question for which you have no answer, ask your instructor during the next class. This brings us to the topic of taking notes.

Whether you are in class or reading alone, there are many ways to take effective notes. The method you use depends on the purpose for the note taking (building vocabulary, memorization of facts, understanding a concept, etc.) and on your style of learning. A few of the most popular note-taking styles are:

- Cornell method: The notebook page is divided into two sections, with the left section approximately 2" wide. Notes are recorded on the right side, and corresponding vocabulary, important concepts, and key words are listed on the left. A brief summary is usually written at the bottom of the page.
- Outline: Topics and subtopics are carefully aligned and indented according to how the information relates to the facts before it. Because of the formal structure of an outline, it is not always the most effective note-taking method for lectures or in-class notes (unless the instructor also uses an outline to teach). While taking "live" notes in class, it may be best not to use the Roman numeral and letter/number format because that makes it impossible to later add important information to the outline; instead, use bullets, dashes, and indentions to mark subtopics.
- Mapping: A central idea, concept, or piece of information is written in the center of the page and corresponding ideas or subtopics are branched out from it via connecting lines. This method is useful when learning a complex concept or theory and is great for visual learners because colors, drawings, or small graphics are easily integrated into the notes.

No matter which methods you use—or if you create your own—there are some important principles to follow to make any note-taking style more effective.

General Guidelines for Note Taking

- Always:
  - Choose a note-taking method that works for your learning style and for the topic.
  - Date and number all your notes.
  - Leave some empty space in case you need to fill in more information later.
- Before class:
  - Read the material thoroughly before class, highlighting important information, making notes in the margin, and indicating questions for the instructor. The class will make much more sense and you'll be ready to ask questions about items that are confusing to you.
  - Write down unfamiliar terms and look them up; make sure you understand the appropriate definition and how it relates to your topic—for example, a crown has a much different meaning to you than it does to a member of royalty.
  - As you take notes, write in your own words, not those of the instructor or textbook. Summarizing, paraphrasing, and even listing information help make sure you understand and internalize the information and make studying and reviewing more user-friendly.
  - Develop and use your own shorthand symbols to later draw your attention to important points (!), questions you have about a point/topic (?), or items that need to be memorized (*). Visual symbols will not only help you quickly locate and identify the material in question *during* class (questions to ask) but also *after* class while reviewing and adding to your notes. The symbols used in the parentheses are simply examples of shorthand symbols. Feel free to be creative or use whatever is most effective for you.
  - Bring your notes and questions to class and review them before class begins.
- During class:
  - Sit where there are the fewest distractions, where you can hear the instructor clearly, and where you can clearly see any notes or demonstrations the instructor provides.
  - Listen for content key words that are specific to the subject. Write down all vocabulary and important facts.
  - Pay attention to clue words and the instructor's physical cues that let you know something important is coming up that you should write down. Some examples of instructor's verbal and nonverbal cues and clues are:
    - "Three important safety regulations . . ." (a list is coming up)
    - "Most importantly . . ."
    - "The advantages and/or disadvantages to this . . ."
    - "First . . . Next . . . Last . . ."
    - Raising the voice or emphasizing words
    - Pointing out items on a chart, in an outline, or even in the text
    - Moving closer to students
    - Repeating words or phrases (sometimes several times)
    - Writing information on the board, overhead transparency, etc.
  - Ask questions. Some instructors ask you to wait until an appointed time, such as after a demonstration or instructional video or even at the end of class, to ask questions.
  - Use common sense. If you are the only one who does not fully understand something, perhaps it's better to wait until after class to ask. Find out what your instructor prefers.
- After class:
  - Review your notes as soon as possible after class, filling in notes, clarifying ideas, and writing down additional questions to ask the instructor or research on your own.
  - Use the shorthand you've developed to point out key terms, important points, confusing concepts, etc.
  - Summarize the notes using just a sentence or two and highlight the summary. It will prove useful when creating a study plan for your exam.

Great note taking will only get you so far. To really know your subject deeply and be able to pass an exam means you also need to review your notes on a regular basis. Regular review helps ensure that you understand the material and cuts down dramatically on the amount of time you'll need to study and review immediately before the exam. After all, you will have been studying all along!

Lastly, use all available tools to check your understanding. Part II of this text contains a content review outline interspersed with review questions. Read through the outline, highlight important information, compare your study notes with the outline, and quiz yourself using the review questions. If you find that you need more preparation in certain areas or that some concepts are still a little vague, go back to your textbook to clarify. After you feel you have mastered the material, use the simulated exam and scoring guide in Part III of this text and on the accompanying CD to test your exam readiness. If you do well, give yourself a well-deserved pat on the back. If you don't perform as well as you had expected, don't despair and don't give up. These are study tools for you to measure your readiness to take the formal exam—they are not end results. Whether you score high, medium, or low on the review questions, use the rationales as an additional tool to better understand any questions you missed and to verify and solidify the correct answers you had. Then make a list and formulate a study plan and schedule to help you focus on the areas in which you had trouble. Remember, studying is a cycle, not a linear process.

Preparing for the Exam

It is very important to prepare yourself physically and psychologically for the exam itself. Arriving at the test center weak, worn out, tired, frazzled, or otherwise unhealthy is not going to help you pass that exam. So what's the best way to prepare? By being proactive, of course!

Avoid Test Anxiety

Many people experience a snowball effect of fear, stress, and anxiety by worrying about how their test anxiety will affect their exam score, increasing their anxiety even more. If you are one of those people, take a deep breath when you catch yourself becoming anxious. Remind yourself that you have been studying and preparing for the test all along. Focus on the positive and build up your confidence instead of tearing it down. Try writing positive messages on sticky notes and posting them around your living space. Be your own cheerleader and recruit family, friends, and fellow students to be your cheerleaders.

Several Days Before the Exam

- Your knowledge of the material should be very solid at this point. Even though you are past the point of learning major new concepts, continue to stick to your study schedule and focus on strengthening any areas in which you feel weak and reviewing those areas in which you are strong. Don't try to memorize the information—own it!
- If you haven't already done so, make flashcards for the various components on the exam. Use the flashcards yourself as a quick check throughout the day or ask supportive family members and friends to quiz you periodically as you have dinner, chat on the phone, etc. Make it a fun game, not a stress-filled obligation.
- Take a practice test—in fact, take more than one. Become familiar with the layout of the exam, the format of the questions, and the wording of the directions. But remember that no practice test can include all the questions on the actual exam or ones similar in phrasing. Study the material, not the specific practice questions.
- Consider completing the DANB online tutorial (available for download at http://www.danb.org/exams/tutorial2.asp) before you get to the test center. It describes how to mark your answers, skip items, and return to questions. You can also take the tutorial at the test site immediately before you begin the test—it does not count toward your testing time. Going through the tutorial twice will ensure you haven't missed anything.
- Get plenty of sleep (at least 6 to 8 hours a night). A tired mind does not function well.
- Try to relax as much as possible and don't spend every waking hour studying. Allow your mind to process all the information you've put into it. If you've done your work all along and internalized the information, the knowledge will be there. Trust in yourself.
- Eat small, nutritious, well-balanced meals several times every day. Feed your body and your mind so you can function at optimal level.

The Day Before the Exam

This is not a time for cramming. You may want to take some time to review, but relaxation and positive attitude building should be your primary concern. If you haven't done so already, drive to the test center at about the same time of day as on the day of the exam in order to judge traffic patterns, time delays, etc. This will help ensure that you allow adequate time to arrive on time at the exam center destination. Locate where you will park, identify the correct entrance, etc. You should also make sure that there is plenty of gas in your vehicle to get you to the location. You do not want to be late, hurried, or confused before you even step foot in the testing center.

The Night Before the Exam

- Have a light, nutritious dinner. You want to make sure you sleep well before the test. Heavy dinners, alcohol, or extremely spicy foods can interfere with a good night's sleep. Avoid them.
- Decide what you will wear. Choose light, comfortable clothing that won't detract your attention. If you get chilled easily, plan to bring a light jacket or sweater.
- Gather the necessary items you'll need to bring with you and place them where you will not forget them on test day:
  - Two forms of valid identification
  - Any additional paperwork you may be required to bring
- Plan to get the optimum amount of sleep for you. For most people, that is between 6 and 8 hours. However, for some, 8 hours can be either too much or not quite enough.
- Check your attitude and build yourself up. This is not a night for cramming or studying. It's a night for relaxing and boosting your confidence.

The Morning of the Exam

At this point, you should be well prepared for the exam. You've laid out your clothes, assembled all required materials, ensured you know how and when to get to the test center, and gotten a good night's rest. All that is left to do is get dressed, eat a light and nutritious breakfast, including some protein, and build up a positive can-do attitude. Leave yourself plenty of time to get to the test center, arriving at least 5 minutes early. If you think better after a morning cup of coffee, then by all means, indulge a little, but be careful not to consume too much caffeine—you don't want to be jittery or anxious—or consume too many liquids. Testing time does not stop while you use the restroom!

During the Exam

As difficult as it may seem, you need to try to relax. Focus on your breathing; don't hold your breath. Also, try to sit in a comfortable, upright position, leaning slightly forward. Being hunched over will only serve to give you a backache and remind you how uncomfortable you are. Don't sit still too long. Move your legs and arms from time to time and rotate your shoulders. Try to keep your blood circulating. Use the tips and strategies provided in the following sections to improve your test-taking abilities.

Tips for Answering Exam Questions

The exam is written using simple multiple-choice questions. This does not mean that the questions themselves are simple, but that the questions are formatted in a simple, straightforward style that *is not* meant to trick or confuse you. However, the exam *is* meant to measure and evaluate your knowledge of the subject. Each question will have only one right answer, along with several "distractor" choices that may look very plausible or even correct at first glance. Distractors are not meant to confuse or trick you, even though it may appear that way at first. Don't allow yourself to become frazzled. Have confidence in your knowledge and read each question and answer carefully. Familiarize yourself with multiple-choice-style questions and follow these strategies when answering multiple-choice questions:

- Read all directions very carefully, even if you think you know what they may say.
- Read the question carefully and look for clues to the right answer:
  - Sometimes, the way a question is phrased will offer a hint by having only one grammatically correct answer.
  - Dissect the question into smaller parts, if possible, to make sure you understand what is being asked.
- Look for words that are capitalized or in bold print in the question. In negative format questions, the words "NOT" or "EXCEPT" indicate that the answer will be negative. The distractors (incorrect answer choices) will be true.
- Look for absolute words in the answer choices, such as "always" or "never," which are rarely the correct answer.
- Have the answer in mind before you begin looking for the correct choice.
- Read each answer choice separately and evaluate whether it answers the question completely, is only part of the right answer, or is completely off topic.

- Eliminate "wrong" answers right away. Just be careful not to do this too quickly; you don't want to eliminate the right answer. Read, evaluate, and think through the choices.
- If you find you really do not know an answer at all, try to eliminate as many of the wrong choices as possible to increase your chances of getting the right answer and then take your best educated guess; you will not be penalized.

Practice using these tips as you answer the review questions in this text and on the accompanying CD.

Strategies for Taking the Exam

- Take the online tutorial available at the test center before you begin your exam, even if you've taken it elsewhere online already.
- Budget your time and don't spend too much time on any one question.
- Conversely, don't hurry. Try to use every bit of time you have available for your exam.
- Use the restroom if necessary, but remember that the timer keeps going even when you're taking a restroom break.
- Don't allow yourself to become frustrated. If you feel anxiety creeping in, take a minute to look away from the computer, take a deep breath, clear your mind, then collect yourself and refocus. Tell yourself you can do this.
- During the exam, you will be able to access a list of commonly used acronyms used on the DANB exam, so don't worry that you'll forget what the letters in OSHA stand for.
- Don't dwell on answers you really don't know. If you truly don't know the right answer, give it your best educated guess and move on. You will not be penalized for guessing incorrectly (some exams will take off more points for wrong answers than blank ones; the DANB does not do this).
- If, after eliminating wrong answers and narrowing down your answer choices, you are still unsure of the correct answer, flag the question for review and come back to it later. Other questions/answer choices may jog your memory and give clues to a previous question.
- Only flag for review the questions where you are really stuck. If you flag too many, you'll likely end up confusing yourself more.
- After you have answered all exam questions within a given component exam, an answer review screen will appear, displaying a comprehensive list of question items and indicating which items you've left blank (incomplete) and which items you've flagged for review or for comment. You may choose to review all items or only review flagged answer choices; however, you must complete your review in the time you have left. You will *not* receive extra exam time to review the answers.
  - If you choose to review all questions, only double-check that you've marked the answer choices that

you *intended*. If you find a mismarked item (for example, you intended to choose answer "A" but somehow marked "C"), change it.

- If you choose to go back to questions you've flagged for review, only change the answer if you find a glaring error. If you are unsure if the answer is right, *do not* second-guess yourself. Leave your first answer. Chances are, your first response is right.
- After the answer review screen, you will be asked to confirm that you are ending the exam review. After you click "yes," you will not be able to return to the exam or change any answers.

■ You may also flag items for comments. After exiting the answer review screen, the comment review screen appears.

- You may choose to comment on all items or only those that you have flagged.
- You are allotted 10 minutes in addition to the exam time for posting comments.
- You cannot change answers or return to answer review mode while in comment review mode.
- After confirming that you are exiting the comment review mode, you cannot return to the exam, to answer review mode, or to comment review mode.

After the Exam

You will receive a preliminary score report at the testing center, and official scores will be mailed to you approximately 4 weeks after your exam. The scores are "scaled," meaning that a complex score is translated into a more user-friendly scale. This scale has a numerical range of 100 (low) to 900 (high). A scaled score of 400 is considered passing for each component. You may retake the component exam(s) that were not passed, but you are required to reapply and pay exam fees for those exams. You must pass all component exams within 5 years to receive certification.

Along with your scaled score, your score report will also show your performance on the subtests or general content areas. The performance indicators will show on which sections you scored "high average" (best), "average" (medium), and "low average" (weak). If you need to retake the test, it is highly recommended that you increase your knowledge in the "low average" subtest material.

For additional information about the DANB exam, such as individualized standards for passing, who else can see your test scores, how you can request a duplicate score report, etc., visit the DANB website at www.danb.org.

GENERAL CHAIRSIDE ASSISTING (GC)

Collecting and Recording Clinical Data

I. Basic Oral and Dental Anatomy and Physiology
  A. Bones of the cranium, face, and neck
    1. Cranial bones are the single frontal, occipital, sphenoid, and ethmoid bones and also the paired parietal and temporal bones.
    2. Facial bones are the lacrimal bones, nasal bones, vomer, nasal conchae, zygomatic bones, maxillae, and mandible.
    3. The hyoid bone is suspended between the mandible and larynx.
  B. Muscles of the head and neck
    1. Muscles of mastication are: temporal muscles, masseter muscles, internal (or medial) pterygoid muscles, and external (or lateral) pterygoid muscles.
    2. Muscles of facial expression are: orbicularis oris muscle, buccinators muscle, mentalis muscle, and zygomatic major.
    3. Muscles of the floor of the mouth are: digastric muscle, mylohyoid muscle, stylohyoid muscle, and geniohyoid muscle.
    4. Muscles of the tongue are classified as intrinsic (within the tongue) or extrinsic (outside the tongue). Intrinsic muscles shape the tongue during speech, mastication, and swallowing. Extrinsic muscles move the tongue.
    5. Muscles of the soft palate (major) are: palatoglossus and palatopharyngeus.
    6. Muscles of the neck are: sternocleidomastoid muscle and trapezius muscle.
  C. Glands
    1. The most significant glands for dental health professionals are the major and minor salivary glands.
    2. The pituitary gland, pineal gland, thyroid gland, and parathyroid glands are found within the head and neck.
    3. The thyroid gland is located within the neck on the front and sides of the trachea just below the larynx.
  D. Nerves
    1. The trigeminal nerve (cranial nerve V) is the primary source of innervation for the oral cavity.
    2. The trigeminal nerve is subdivided into three divisions: maxillary, mandibular, and ophthalmic. Of these three divisions, the maxillary and mandibular are of particular interest to dental health professionals.
  E. Blood vessels
    1. Major arteries of the face and mouth are the aorta and the common carotid artery.
    2. Blood descends from the face and mouth through this network of veins: maxillary vein, temporal vein, retromandibular vein, and lingual veins. These veins empty into the jugular veins, which empty into the superior vena cava to transport blood to the heart and lungs for reoxygenation.

    F. Teeth
1. There are essentially four components of the tooth: enamel, dentin, pulp, and cementum.
2. The tooth consists of a crown and a root.
    a. The anatomic crown of the tooth is the part covered by enamel. The *clinical crown* refers to the part of the crown visible in the oral cavity.
    b. The anatomic root is the part of the tooth covered by cementum. The *clinical root* refers only to the part of the root that is not visible.

    G. Oral cavity
1. The vestibule is the space between the teeth and the inner lining of the cheeks and lips.
2. The frena (singular: frenum), raised lines of mucosal tissue, are visible when the lips are pulled back and they support or restrain teeth and other structures.
3. The gingivae—commonly called the gums—are attached to the alveolar ridge and vary in color from pale pink to brownish pink. *Free gingivae* or *marginal gingivae* is where the gingivae meet the teeth and is the first area to respond to inflammation.
4. The hard palate, a bony plate covered with keratinized tissue, sits toward the front of the mouth and forms the anterior portion of the palate.
5. The soft palate is composed of muscle tissue rather than bone and sits toward the back of the mouth. The uvula, the projection visible when the mouth is opened wide, hangs from the back of the soft palate.

II. Clinical Exam
    A. While escorting patient to the clinical examination area, observe patient's overall appearance, gait, speech, and general behavior and note unusual or concerning characteristics or behavior.
    B. Seat patient upright in dental chair, secure paper bib or napkin around patient's neck, and compile or update patient's medical and dental history. Note drug allergies and chronic diseases, such as diabetes; record the purpose of the patient's visit.
    C. Types and locations of teeth in the primary and permanent dentition
1. Incisors cut food, support lips, and help produce sounds for speech.
2. There are four canine teeth (cuspids), one in each quadrant of the mouth. They have a single cusp (cingulum), whose primary purpose is to tear food.
3. Premolars are found only in the permanent dentition. They replace the first and second molars of the primary dentition.
4. First and second molars have four cusps used to chew and grind food.
5. Third molars ("wisdom" teeth) erupt in late adolescence/early adulthood.
    D. Surfaces of the tooth are: facial, lingual, incisal/occlusal, mesial, and distal. They are named for their relationship or closeness to other intraoral structures, such as the lips and tongue, or according to which direction they face within the intraoral cavity.
    E. Record abnormal findings in head and neck (TMJ) region
1. As the dentist comments on the patient's dental conditions and health, note or chart any abnormalities, such as: soft tissue abnormalities; tooth structure abnormalities, including missing teeth; and restorations.
2. If allowed in your state, examine extraoral soft tissue by palpation. When searching for oral cancer, examine the head and neck, including inspection and palpation of extraoral tissues, temporomandibular joint, tongue, floor of mouth, palate, uvula, and lymph nodes.
3. Note any other abnormal findings in the head or neck region that may be related to other health conditions.

III. Patient Charts
    A. Identify permanent and primary teeth using numbering systems
1. The universal numbering system is the main numbering system used on dental charts in the United States.
2. The international tooth numbering system is a two-digit system that uses only numerals 1 through 8 for each digit.
3. The Palmer notation system identifies the teeth by quadrant and number.
    B. Chart conditions
1. Use Black's classification of cavities (describes six classes of cavities and outlines restorative treatments for each) to observe/record suspected cavities.
2. Use abbreviations, symbols, and colors in the patient chart to document decay, restoration, or other existing conditions.

3. Record the results of the periodontal exam, including the dentist's assessment of mobility, pocket depth, and furcation involvement.

4. Record existing damage or disease to tooth pulp (endodontics) or periapical tissue.

IV. Diagnostic Testing

  A. Assist in collecting diagnostic patient information.

1. Dental radiographs allow the dentist to examine the health of the pulp, the root canal space, and the bone and to detect possible dental caries.

2. Various pulp tests, such as thermal pulp testing and electric pulp testing, are used to diagnose periodontal disease.

3. Photography can provide a before-and-after record of original conditions and the subsequent effects of any procedures.

4. Preparing materials for taking an occlusal registration include (1) softening the wax in warm water and preparing it for placement in the patient's mouth and (2) mixing other materials on a paper pad and putting them on a quadrant tray for placement in the patient's mouth.

  B. Diagnostic casts (diagnostic models or study models) are three-dimensional models of the patient's teeth, mouth, and arches. They are useful because they show actual distances and proportion of the patient's teeth and arches. They are created from alginate impressions and included in the patient's record.

V. Documenting Treatment

  A. Maintain accurate records of drugs prescribed or dispensed to patients. If a drug is discussed in detail with the patient, record important points of this discussion.

  B. Before the patient arrives, familiarize yourself with the patient's record to alert you to the patient's premedications (premeds), any medical concerns you and the dental team should be aware of, any change in dental treatment that should be provided, and any change in the way in which dental treatments should be performed.

  C. Record recommended treatment in patient's chart and make sure the chart includes signed and dated consent forms necessary for treatment. If a patient refuses an examination, treatment, or test, document the refusal in the chart. If possible, ask the patient to sign a statement indicating that they refused treatment and keep that statement in the chart.

  D. Record that the patient complied with the treatment provided.

VI. Obtain Vital Signs

  A. Take a pulse by gently palpating an artery with fingertips, pressing lightly but firmly enough to feel the pulse. Count the number of pulse beats for 30 seconds; multiply your count by two and record pulse rate in patient chart, along with date, time, and your signature.

  B. Measure respiration by counting the number of times the patient's chest rises and falls in 30 seconds. Each cycle of rise and fall of the chest counts as one. Multiply your count by two and record respiration rate in patient chart, along with date, time, and your signature.

  C. Measure blood pressure using a sphygmomanometer and a stethoscope. Record blood pressure in patient chart, along with date, time, and your signature. The systolic number is written first, followed by the diastolic.

  D. Temperature is measured with a thermometer at different body sites: under the tongue, inside the armpit, inside the ear, and inside the rectum (for infants). Record temperature in patient chart, along with date, time, and your signature.

Review Questions

1. Using the universal numbering system, the permanent maxillary right second molar is tooth number
   A. 2.
   B. 7.
   C. 15.
   D. 18.

2. A small, rounded extension of bone covered with soft tissue located posterior to the last maxillary molar is the
    A. Stensen's papilla.
    B. retromolar pad.
    C. maxillary tuberosity.
    D. torus palatinus.

3. Which of the following best describes the palantine rugae?
    A. The demarcation between the hard and soft palate.
    B. Horizontally raised folds of hard tissue behind the incisive papilla on the hard palate.
    C. The ridged line that extends from behind the incisive papilla down the midline of the palate.
    D. A raised area of tissue just behind the maxillary incisors.

4. To identify Stensen's papilla, look for a
    A. small raised flap of soft tissue on the buccal mucosa opposite the maxillary second molar.
    B. triangular area of bone covered with soft tissue behind the last mandibular molar.
    C. raised horizontal extension of soft tissue along the occlusal line on the buccal mucosa.
    D. raised rounded area of soft tissue directly behind the two maxillary central incisors.

5. Which of the following nerves provides sensory innervation for the teeth and mouth?
    A. Trapezius
    B. Glossopharyngeal
    C. Trigeminal
    D. Zygomatic

6. Which of the following major salivary glands is located on the side of the face, behind the ramus, below and in front of the ear?
    A. Buccal
    B. Parotid
    C. Sublingual
    D. Submandibular

See p. 33 for the correct answers and rationales

General Dentistry Chairside Procedures

I. Assisting with the Patient and Equipment

    A. Prepare the treatment room by cleaning and disinfecting clinical contact areas; placing infection control barriers in the area; bringing the patient's record, radiographs, and lab work to the area; bringing in a sterile preset tray and other supplies; clearing a pathway for the patient; and positioning the dental chair.

    B. Prepare treatment trays by lining up instruments in the order in which they'll be used. Place those instruments to be used first on the left side of the tray and hinged instruments on the right side of the tray. Also, arrange instruments and material based on their function.

    C. Greet the patient in the reception area and invite him or her to the treatment room. Once seated in the dental chair, position the patient upright, supine, semisupine, or subsupine (Trendelenburg). Position yourself, the operator, the dental unit, and all instruments and equipment that will be needed during a procedure so that you and the operator use only class I, II, and III motions.

    D. Four-handed dentistry, or team dentistry, is the method of providing dental treatment in which the operator and assistant work together as a team while both are seated in specific positions near the patient.

        1. Maintain the dentist's fulcrum during instrument transfer. A fulcrum is a hand position in which the dentist's fingers are stabilized so the hand can easily pivot and perform work in the oral cavity.

        2. Sit across from the dentist and hand instruments across the transfer zone to the dentist as needed. The transfer zone is the space where instrument transfer occurs during four-handed dentistry, usually below the patient's chin and directly over his or her throat and upper chest.

3. After the patient has been placed in the proper position, the chair may need to be raised or lowered by the operator to get a clear vision of the operating field and to allow ergonomic access to the oral cavity.

II. Select and Prepare Trays and Other Dental Equipment

A. Select, prepare, and modify impression trays.

1. Selecting a proper tray from among a supply of stock trays requires that you try several before choosing one that causes the patient as little discomfort as possible.

2. Modify stock trays with utility wax. If a stock tray does not fit a patient's needs, construct custom trays, which are specially designed and built to fit a particular patient's mouth. Several types of materials may be used, which may be self-curing or light-cured acrylic resin, vacuum resin, or a thermoplastic material.

B. The tray for local anesthetic administration should include aspirating syringe, two carpules of anesthetic, long and short needles, alcohol sponge, cotton gauze, tongue depressor (optional), needle recapping device, sharps disposal system, topical anesthetic, and a cotton applicator on a clean cotton gauze.

C. Select and prepare tray setups and equipment.

1. The tray setup for anesthetics varies depending on the type of anesthetic being administered.
   a. Topical anesthetics setups require a topical agent, gauze pad, and applicator.
   b. Local anesthetics require injection equipment and an anesthetic cartridge.
   c. Inhalation anesthesia requires nitrous oxide and oxygen cylinders and related equipment.
   d. Intravenous sedation setup requires an antiseptic, small needle, tourniquet, and IV.

2. Permanent restorations require a restorative tray (basic setup, hand-cutting instruments, amalgam carrier, condensers, burnishers, carvers, composite placement instrument, articulating paper holder), local anesthetic setup, dental dam setup, high-volume oral evacuator tip, high-speed handpiece, low-speed handpiece, saliva ejector, burs, cotton pellets and rolls, gauze, dental liners, base, bonding agents, sealers, permanent restorative material (composite or amalgam), and dental floss.

3. Tray setup for tooth whitening includes basic setup, protective gel or dental dam, tooth whitener product, resin polishing cup or fluoride prophy paste, and a light or laser source.

4. Crown setups require cotton rolls, bite stick, plastic filling instrument, permanent luting cement, scaler or explorer, custom fabricated crown, and cementing materials.

5. Bridge setups need cotton rolls, petroleum jelly, alginate impression, self-curing acrylic resin with spatula and mixing container, finishing diamonds or burs, rubber wheels and cusp for polishing, polishing paste, and cementing materials.

6. Cotton rolls or gauze, a microbrush, and a desensitizing agent are needed for desensitization.

7. Root canal procedures require a local anesthetic agent setup (optional), dental dam setup, handpiece (high speed) with burs, handpiece (low speed) with latch attachment, syringe, broaches and Hedstrom/K-type files of assorted lengths/sizes, rubber instrument stops, lentulo spiral, paper points, gutta-percha points, spoon excavator, endodontic explorer, endodontic sealer supplies, Glick #1, locking cotton pliers, millimeter ruler, sodium hypochlorite solution, hemostat, and high-volume oral evacuator (HVE) tip.

8. Pupal therapies require local anesthetic agent setup, dental dam setup, low-speed handpiece, round burs, spoon excavators, sterile cotton pellets, formocresol, zinc oxide eugenol base, final restorative material, and instruments for placement.

9. The exact composition of the surgical tray setup for extractions, impactions, incisions and drainage, prosthetic implants, and suture placement and removal depends on the procedure and operator, so it's essential to understand the nature of the surgery and the surgeon's preferences while assembling the setup.

10. Partial dentures require a basic tray setup, complete with mouth mirror, explorer, and cotton pliers; articulating paper and forceps; pressure indicator paste; a low-speed handpiece and acrylic and finishing burs; three-pronged pliers; and the patient's partial denture.

11. Full and immediate denture setups require a mouth mirror, explorer, and cotton pliers; HVE and air-water syringe tips; a hand mirror; articulating forceps and paper; high-speed and low-speed handpieces and burs and discs; the patient's dentures from the laboratory; and take-home materials and hygiene aids.

12. Fluoride treatments require disposable applicator trays, a saliva ejector, air-water syringe, cotton rolls, and a timer.

13. Initial impressions for partial and full dentures require a basic tray setup and stock trays for alginate impressions and a wax bite registration. The alginate impressions will be used to make the custom trays used in the secondary impressions.

14. Secondary impressions for partial dentures require the basic tray setup, mouth wash, the custom tray created for the patient or a stock tray, contouring wax and impression materials (spatula and mixing pad or dispensing gun and tips), a laboratory prescription form, disinfectant, wax or silicone bite registration materials, a container for the impressions and bite registration, and tooth shade and mold guides.

15. Secondary impression setups for full dentures require a mouth mirror, explorer, and cotton pliers; HVE and air-water syringe tips; cotton rolls and gauze; mouthwash; the patient's custom tray; compound wax and a Bunsen burner; laboratory knife; impression materials; laboratory prescription form; disinfectant; and a container for the impressions and bite registration.

16. Setups for fixed space maintainer appliances require permanent cement, a mouth mirror and explorer, cotton roll and gauze, HVE and air-water syringe, an appliance from laboratory, and articulation paper.

17. Occlusal equilibration/adjustment requires a mouth mirror, articulation paper, high-speed and low-speed handpieces, and burs and discs.

18. Oral examination setups require a mouth mirror, explorer, cotton pliers, periodontal probe, gauze sponges/squares, dental floss, articulating paper and paper holder, air-water syringe, red and blue colored pencils, eraser, and a clean, unmarked examination form clipped to the patient chart.

19. Oral prophylaxis tray setup includes a mouth mirror, explorer, cotton gauze and swabs, low-speed handpiece, rubber cups and brushes, prophy paste, and dental floss.

20. Periodontal procedure setups, such as scaling and polishing, require a mouth mirror, explorer, probe, scalers and curettes, gauze, dental floss and tape, prophy angle with rubber cups and brushes, and prophy paste.

21. Surgical periodontal procedure setups, such as gingivectomy, require a mouth mirror, explorer, cotton pliers, periodontal probe, cotton rolls and gauze sponges, saliva ejector with tips, markers, periodontal knives, scalpel, blades, burs, scalers and curettes, soft tissue rongeurs, surgical scissors, hemostat, suture supplies, anesthestic supplies, and periodontal dressing supplies.

22. Surgical dressing placement setups require a mouth mirror, explorer, cotton pliers, gauze sponges, dressing material, paper pad, tongue depressor, lubricant, and contouring instrument.

23. Surgical dressing removal setups require a mouth mirror, explorer, cotton pliers, spoon excavator, suture scissors, floss, saliva ejector with various tips, gauze sponges, and tissue.

24. Root planing and curettage setups require the mouth mirror, explorer, probe, scalers, curettes, gauze, dental floss and tape, prophy angle with rubber cups and brushes, and prophy paste.

25. Dental dams require sheets of pliable, thin latex or latex-free material; frames; napkins; lubricants; templates and stamps; punch; clamps; forceps; floss; and stabilization cord.

26. Dental sealants require protective eyeware, rubber dam or cotton balls, sealant material, etching agent gel or liquid, pumice and water, prophy brush, applicator device or syringe, high-volume oral evacuator, curing light with shield, articulating paper and holder, low-speed dental handpiece with contra-angle attachment, and round white stone (latch type).
    a. Temporary crown setup requires cotton rolls, bite stick, plastic filling instrument, temporary luting cement, scaler or explorer, and prefabricated crown
    b. Temporary restorations require a Tofflemire matrix retainer (for class II), a matrix band system (for classes II, III, and IV), a wedge (for classes II, III, and IV), intermediate restoration material setup, condenser, carvers, discoid/cleoid, plastic instrument, carver, Hollenback, cotton pellet, and articulating paper.
    c. The basic setup for dry socket or alveolitis requires a mouth mirror, explorer, cotton pliers, periodontal probe, cotton rolls and gauze sponges, saliva ejector with tips, HVE, scissors, irrigation solution, warm saline solution, iodoform gauze, and medicated dressing.
    d. Rotary instruments

III. Assisting with and Performing Intraoral Procedures
    A. Maintain the field of operation.
        1. Keep the operating field well lit, free from debris and moisture, and easily accessible. Move obstructing tissues out of the line of vision with instruments such as tissue retractors.
        2. Use an air-water syringe in conjunction with the HVE to remove saliva, blood, and debris from the oral cavity.
        3. Clean the area around the operating field with either limited rinsing or complete oral rinsing.
        4. Use cotton rolls, dry angle, or rubber dam to isolate the area.

B. Place and remove cotton rolls with gloved fingers or cotton pliers.
C. Assisting with or polishing the teeth.
   1. Begin with the surface of the tooth closest to the cheek (the buccal surface) and proceed from the right side of the mouth to the left, moving across the mandibular arch.
   2. After all of the mandibular teeth are polished, work proceeds from left to right, focusing on the side of the teeth closest to the tongue.
   3. Next, the teeth of the maxillary arch are polished in the same order and manner. Utilizing a low-speed handpiece and a prophy angle, and the finest grit prophylaxis paste possible, the teeth should be polished using a light, intermittent pressure for 1 to 2 seconds per tooth.
D. Apply topical fluoride, which is available in gels and foams.
   1. Remove all plaque and calculus.
   2. Seat the patient upright throughout the procedure with a saliva ejector placed between the arches to prevent ingestion of fluoride.
   3. Select a fluoride tray.
   4. After loading the fluoride into the tray, dry the teeth and insert the tray into the patient's mouth.
   5. Instruct the patient to bite down to spread the fluoride throughout the teeth.
   6. Set the timer and stay with the patient throughout the treatment.
   7. After the timer has ended, remove excess saliva and fluoride from the oral cavity.
E. To perform vitality tests, use palpation, percussion, thermal testing, electric testing, radiography, or transillumination testing.
F. After surgery, control minor bleeding with cotton or gauze pads.
G. Assist with the placement and removal of temporary cement.
H. After a temporary crown is cemented, remove the extra cement from the edge of the tooth with the dental explorer. Use floss to remove cement from between teeth.
I. Place dental dams after the dentist administers the anesthetic and remove the dental dam after the procedure.
   1. Make sure the site is free from plaque and debris.
   2. Mark the dental dam for the appropriate teeth and punch the keyhole and the holes for individual teeth. Each hole should be separated by a slight septum that will be eased into the interproximal space.
   3. Select a clamp and tie a safety line of dental floss to the clamp bow. Grip the clamp with the forceps, spread the beaks of the forceps, and use the sliding bar to hold them open. Place the clamp by sliding it over the anchor tooth. Gently release the forceps and remove the beaks from the anchor holes.
   4. If you haven't already placed the dental dam, slide the keyhole over the clamp's bow. Retrieve the dental floss ligature with cotton pliers or an explorer and slide it through the dental dam. Secure the dental dam to the opposite tooth.
   5. Place the dental napkin around the patient's oral cavity and slide the frame into position. Hook the dental dam material on the frame to hold it steady.
   6. Work the remaining teeth to be isolated through the punched holes in the dental dam material.
   7. Work the dental dam septum in between the tooth contacts, using floss if necessary to ensure that the dental dam is located below the contacts.
   8. Remove the dental dam when indicated. To remove the dental dam, first remove the clamp and any ligature or stabilization cord used to secure the dental dam. Pull the dental dam away from the teeth. Clip the interseptal dam bridges. Then remove the dam and frame in one motion. Inspect the dental dam to make sure no part was left inside the patient's mouth.
J. Prepare, assist with, and/or apply a matrix band and remove the matrix band after the procedure.
   1. Select the band and contour it to make sure it is thinned and slightly concave.
   2. Place the band into the retainer handle and insert the retainer into the oral cavity, parallel to the buccal surface.
   3. Slide the open band down over the occlusal surface of the tooth.
   4. Adjust the inner knob until the band has tightened around the tooth. Make sure the band is adapted to the tooth surface and there is no material or tissue between the band and the tooth.
   5. Remove the matrix band when indicated.
K. To apply a topical ointment, dry the site with a gauze pad. Then place a small amount of the anesthetic on the injection site for several minutes.

L. Assist with and/or monitor the administration of nitrous oxide.
   1. Sedation with nitrous oxide begins and ends with giving the patient pure O_2.
   2. At the start of the process, the clinician establishes the patient's tidal volume and then slowly titrates the concentration of N_2O until the appropriate level is achieved.
   3. At the end of the sedation process, 100% O_2 should be given again, for several minutes. Ask the patient about symptoms such as dizziness, headache, or tiredness. When the patient reports feeling normal, check vital signs again.
M. Rotary instruments, such as burs and abrasive instruments, can include tips for cutting, grinding, polishing, and abrading dental surfaces.
   1. Burs are available in different shapes (e.g., round, cone, etc.) and in different materials (e.g., diamond, steel, etc.). Burs are typically identified by their structure and form, as well as their length.
   2. Abrasive instruments are most often used to finish restorations, although some can be used for cutting. They lack cutting blades, but instead feature a variety of abrasive materials on a variety of bases and shapes. Abrasive instruments are classified by their shape (e.g., wheel, disc, etc.) and their material (e.g., rubber, stone, etc.).
   3. Exchange the rotary instrument in the dental handpiece as needed.
N. Assist with general dentistry and dental emergencies.
   1. Anesthesia includes topical and local anesthetics.
      a. To apply a topical ointment, dry the site with a gauze pad, place a small amount of the anesthetic on a cotton-tipped applicator and place it on the injection site, holding it in place for several minutes before the injection is administered.
      b. The dental assistant assembles and passes the syringe to the clinician, receives the syringe after injection, and recaps using the scoop or one-handed method. The oral cavity is rinsed and the dental assistant remains with the patient while the local anesthetic takes effect.
   2. In cavity preparation and restoration, be familiar with the differences between the various kinds of restorations, including the instrumentation used in each procedure, the materials required, and the dentist's and patient's needs during the procedure. Your role depends on the specific legal requirements and regulations of your state. In states with expanded functions, you may place bases, liners, and varnishes or create temporary restorations. In states without this function, you will help the dentist perform these tasks.
   3. Assist in crown and bridge restoration preparation, temporization, and cementation.
      a. Crowns
         1. Before a crown can be placed, the area of the tooth just under the gingival tissue must be exposed with a retraction cord.
         2. Prepare the impression material. Load the resin into the prepared impression and transfer the impression to the dentist, who makes the impression and places the provisional crown.
         3. After the provisional crown is removed, assist the dentist in placing the permanent crown by rinsing and drying the tooth and surrounding it with cotton rolls. Then mix the permanent cement and transfer it to the dentist, who places the permanent crown.
      b. Bridges
         1. Place and remove the gingival cord so an accurate impression can be taken, which helps ensure the provisional bridge is fabricated to the correct size.
         2. To make a provisional bridge, first make an impression of the teeth and arch. Then mix the resin and place it onto the impression so the dentist can place it in the patient's oral cavity. After the resin sets for a few minutes, the dentist removes it from the patient's mouth. Carefully remove the provisional coverage from the impression. The dentist then places it back into the patient's mouth while it continues to set.
         3. The dentist marks and trims off excess material and attaches the provisional bridge with temporary cement.
   4. To desensitize teeth, the dental assistant dries the sensitive tooth with a cotton roll or gauze and hands the desensitizing agent and microbrush to the dentist to apply.
   5. The two common endodontic therapies are a root canal and a pulpotomy.
      a. For a root canal, aid in preparation by taking a radiograph of the tooth and placing rubber stops on the endodontic files and reamers for the correct filling of the canal. Isolate the tooth being treated by assisting with preparation and placement of the dental dam and clean the area to be treated with disinfectant and a cotton swab.

   b. For a pulpotomy, prepare and place the dental dam and clean the area to be treated with disinfectant and a cotton swab. After the pulp chamber is exposed by the dentist, transfer a spoon excavator to the dentist for removal of pulp tissue in the coronal chamber. To control hemorrhaging, transfer to the dentist a sterile cotton pellet moistened with formocresol for placement in the pulp chamber.

6. Assist with extractions and impactions.
   a. For a simple tooth extraction, prepare the patient for surgery and administer a topical anesthetic and assist in the administration of a local anesthetic. Transfer the elevator and forceps to the surgeon as he or she performs the extraction. Be ready to remove blood and debris and adjust the light during the procedure. To assist with tissue retraction, place a pad of gauze in the empty socket to stop bleeding.
   b. In the case of impacted teeth, or complex extractions, first assist the surgeon with anesthesia. During the operation, transfer instruments to the surgeon and use a special surgical suction tip to prevent surgical complications. During suturing, place the sutures in the needle holder and retract the cheeks.

7. Assist with partial and full dentures.
   a. In fabricating a partial denture, help with the final impression, wax-denture try-in, and placement of the denture.
   b. In fabricating a full denture, help with the final impression and placement of a full denture.

8. Assist the dentist with occlusal equilibration/adjustment.

9. When assisting with an occlusal registration, have the patient open and close his or her mouth several times and observe the patient's normal pattern. Have the patient rinse to remove debris. Then place the cold wax over the occlusal and incisal surfaces of the teeth. If the wax is long enough, trim away extra length. Soften the wax and place it against the surfaces of the teeth. Have the patient bite gently. After the wax hardens, remove it from the patient's mouth.

10. Carefully observe the oral examination conducted by the dentist. As the dentist comments on the patient's dental conditions and health, note or chart the findings on specially designed forms for the patient's record.

11. The prophylaxis angle, or prophy angle, is an angled instrument that holds the rubber cup or brush bristles used for oral prophylaxis. When using the prophy angle and handpiece, the operator alternates between lighter and heavier pressure and applies strokes in a circular motion. Steady pressure can cause excess heat, which can damage the tooth and cause pain for the patient. The foot pedal should be released as soon as the prophy angle and handpiece is no longer touching the tooth; otherwise, it can cause the polishing material to splatter.

12. Periodontal procedures can be either nonsurgical, such as scaling and polishing, or surgical, such as a gingivectomy.
   a. Assist with periodontal procedures by providing retraction of the patient's lips, tongue, and cheek and transferring instruments as needed.
   b. A dry field is maintained with the high-velocity evacuator to remove excess oral fluids.
   c. If periodontal dressing is needed, it is prepared and passed to the dentist.
   d. Periodontal dressing removal is accomplished at the postoperative visit.

13. Apply dental sealants.
   a. First clean and rinse the teeth.
   b. Then isolate the teeth and make sure they are dry. Isolation is usually achieved with a dental dam or cotton rolls.
   c. Apply the etchant to the tooth enamel and remove with suction and rinse the remainder away.
   d. Dry the enamel and apply a sealant with a syringe or brush. If necessary, cure the sealant.
   e. Check coverage with a mouth mirror.

14. Assist with perioperative treatment and complications.

15. Assist with dental implants and bone grafts.
   a. Dental implants may take place in one-stage or two-stage surgeries. Assist with anesthesia, placement of template over the implants, and transfer the cleaned implant and instruments to the doctor. Irrigation and evacuation of the surgical field is maintained throughout the procedure.
   b. During a bone graft, help to maintain ease of visibility, rinse the patient's mouth, transfer instruments as needed for shaping and contouring, and prepare sutures.

16. Assist with suture placement and removal.
    a. To assist in placing sutures, first remove sterile suture material, and using a needle holder, hold the needle in the upper third, away from the sharp point. Transfer the needle holder to the surgeon and provide tissue retraction during placement of the sutures. After the sutures are tied, cut the sutures with suture scissors.
    b. To assist in removing sutures, transfer the cotton pliers to the oral surgeon to lift away the suture and expose the knot. Transfer suture scissors to surgeon to cut sutures. Retract tissues as necessary. Keep track of the number of sutures removed and compare it to the dental record to make sure they are all removed.
17. Assist in taking impressions.
    a. When assisting with an impression, first prepare the basic tray setup.
    b. As the dentist prepares and places the impression material in the tray, prepare materials for taking the bite registration: softening the wax in warm water and preparing it for placement in the patient's mouth.
    c. Mix the other materials on a paper pad and put them on a quadrant tray for placement in the patient's mouth.
    d. After these materials have set, remove them.
    e. Disinfect the impressions.
IV. Working with Patients
    A. Communicate in a way that conveys professionalism, care, and concern. Focus on office procedures, policies, and patient care. Try to understand patients' thoughts and feelings in order to help patients feel calm and relaxed.
    B. Strive to maximize the well-being and health of every patient. This goal can involve extra effort when patients have special needs, such as physical or intellectual disabilities. Patients who have special needs may require extra assistance.
    C. The best way to prepare for, or prevent, a medical emergency is to be alert and gather as much information as possible, including a thorough medical history. Monitor patients who are taking drugs (both pharmaceutical and illicit drugs) more closely.

Review Questions

7. In rubber dam placement, the purpose of inverting the dam is to
    A. stabilize the restoration.
    B. remove excess material.
    C. prevent the clamp from slipping.
    D. prevent saliva leakage.

8. Which of the following instruments is likely to be included in a basic tray setup?
    A. Chisel
    B. Mouth mirror
    C. Angle former
    D. Amalgam carrier

9. A carious lesion in a pit or a fissure would be classified as:
    A. Class I caries: a lesion located in a pit or fissure of a tooth.
    B. Class II caries: a lesion located in the interproximal surfaces of a posterior tooth (premolar or molar).
    C. Class III caries: a lesion located in the interproximal area of anterior teeth such as canines or incisors.
    D. Class V caries: a lesion located on the cervical area of the tooth.

10. Which of the following is an example of biological pulpal stimuli?
    A. Changes from hot and cold coming into contact with the tooth
    B. Changes in occlusion, resulting in trauma
    C. Acidic materials coming into contact with pulpal tissues
    D. Bacteria from saliva coming into contact with pulpal tissues

11. What does an etchant remove in preparation for dental bonding?
    A. Resin veneer
    B. Dentinal tubules
    C. Smear layer
    D. Pulp

12. Which of the following procedures uses enamel bonding?
    A. Sealant
    B. Dental varnish
    C. Calcium hydroxide
    D. Dental base

13. Which instrument is used first during an amalgam restoration?
    A. Excavator
    B. Cleoid-discoid
    C. Burnisher
    D. Condenser

14. Which one of the following tests provides a definitive diagnosis of oral cancer?
    A. Bleeding upon probing
    B. Checking mucosal and gingival pallor
    C. Running laboratory blood tests
    D. Performing a biopsy

15. Which of the following may help prevent a patient from gagging during an alginate impression?
    A. Storing the alginate in a humid environment
    B. Using warm water to mix the alginate
    C. Mixing the alginate slowly
    D. Adding an accelerant to the alginate

16. The curing time of composite restorations depends on the
    A. shade of the restorative material.
    B. age of the restorative material.
    C. etching time.
    D. rinsing time.

17. Which of the following must be done first when preparing a tooth for provisional coverage?
    A. Placement of gingival retraction cord
    B. Preliminary impression
    C. Placement of the post and core
    D. Removal of tooth structure

18. When assisting during final impressions in a crown and bridge preparation, which elastomeric impression material is applied first to the teeth?
    A. Light-bodied
    B. Regular-bodied
    C. Heavy-bodied
    D. Extra heavy-bodied

19. What is the operating zone for an assistant who is assisting a right-handed operator?
    A. 12 o'clock to 2 o'clock
    B. 2 o'clock to 4 o'clock
    C. 4 o'clock to 7 o'clock
    D. 7 o'clock to 12 o'clock

20. Which part of an anesthetic syringe locks into the rubber stopper so that the stopper can be retracted by pulling back on the piston rod?
    A. Barrel
    B. Thumb ring
    C. Piston rod
    D. Harpoon

21. During a class II amalgam procedure, when is the wedge removed?
    A. Before the matrix band and holder are removed
    B. After the matrix band and holder are removed
    C. Before placement of the amalgam
    D. After placement of the amalgam

22. When preparing a Tofflemire matrix band and retainer, the inner nut on the retainer is used to
    A. tighten the spindle within the diagonal slot vise.
    B. loosen the spindle within the diagonal slot vise.
    C. adjust the size of the matrix band loop.
    D. hold the wedge in place.

23. Using the clock concept, the zone located between 4 o'clock and 7 o'clock when working with a right-handed operator is the
    A. assistant's zone.
    B. operator's zone.
    C. static zone.
    D. transfer zone.

24. When an instrument is held in the palm of the hand with all four fingers surrounding the instrument and the thumb supporting the instrument, which grasp is being used?
    A. Pen
    B. Modified pen
    C. Palm
    D. Palm-thumb

25. When passing an instrument that will be used on tooth number 17, the working end should be in what position?
    A. Upward toward the maxillary teeth
    B. Downward toward the mandibular teeth
    C. Facing to the right
    D. Facing to the left

26. Which of the following medications could increase the patient's blood pressure and heart rate?
    A. Aspirin
    B. Warfarin
    C. Over-the-counter cold medication
    D. Nitroglycerin

27. In the United States, nitrous oxide tanks are color-coded
    A. green.
    B. white.
    C. blue.
    D. orange.

28. The drug of choice for dental and outpatient inflammatory pain is
    A. aspirin.
    B. morphine.
    C. acetaminophen.
    D. ibuprofen.

29. Which drug would be contraindicated in patients with peptic ulcers?
    A. Aspirin
    B. Acetaminophen
    C. Morphine
    D. Codeine

30. Nitrous oxide/oxygen inhalation is indicated for which of the following conditions?
    A. Adenoid obstruction
    B. Dental anxiety
    C. Nasal deformity
    D. Bronchitis

31. Codeine is classified at what level of abuse and addiction potential?
    A. Schedule I
    B. Schedule II
    C. Schedule III
    D. Schedule IV

32. Why would an oral surgeon administer diazepam (Valium) to a patient before extraction of a molar?
    A. To reduce postoperative nausea
    B. To relieve anxiety
    C. To increase metabolism
    D. To control muscle movement

33. What is the most commonly used formulation of topical anesthetic?
    A. 20% lidocaine
    B. 5% lidocaine
    C. 5% benzocaine
    D. 20% benzocaine

See p. 33 for the correct answers and rationales

Preparing and Working with Chairside Materials

I. Impressions
   A. Prepare various materials for impressions.
      1. To mix irreversible hydrocolloid (alginate), measure and place water and alginate powder into the bowl. Mix with the spatula until smooth. After mixing, fill the impression tray. Alginate impressions should be poured with model material within 1 hour of being taken to prevent distortion.
      2. Reversible hydrocolloid is an impression material that changes physical states upon heating and cooling.
         a. A stock water-cooled tray is selected to fit the patient's mouth without impinging on soft tissues or teeth.
         b. To prevent sticking, plastic stops are placed in the tray.
         c. Tubing is connected to the tray and the water outlet to drain.
         d. Warm water is pumped through the tubing and tray to liquefy and then moved to a second storage bath.
         e. Light-bodied material is placed in a syringe, heavy-bodied material is placed in the tray, and the tray is moved to the third tempering bath.

f. Light-bodied material is placed around the prepared tooth and the dentist seats the tray.

g. The water running through the tray and tubing is cooled to solidify the impression.

3. Elastomeric materials include polysulfide and silicone. To mix these impressions, dispense equal lengths of the base and catalyst onto the mixing pad and mix with spatula until the color is uniform. Load material into impression tray and deliver to the dentist.

4. To prepare bitewing wax, place the cold wax over the occlusal and incisal surfaces of the teeth. If the wax is long enough, trim away extra length. Soften the wax and place it against the surfaces of the teeth. Have the patient bite gently. After the wax hardens, remove it from the patient's mouth.

II. Restorative Materials

A. Prepare various materials for restorations.

1. Amalgam

a. To prepare amalgam, place the mercury and alloy capsule in an activator, if needed, to break the membrane separating the two materials.

b. Then place the capsule in an amalgamator or triturator to mix the mercury and alloy.

c. After it emerges from the amalgamator, the amalgam is ready to be loaded into the amalgam carrier, according to the dentist's preference.

d. Store mercury and amalgam scraps according to local ordinances, or submerged in a covered, unbreakable container filled with used X-ray fixer.

2. Form dental cement by mixing a powder and liquid, which causes a chemical reaction. Mix cements on either a glass mixing slab or mixing paper with a spatula, following the manufacturer's instructions. The assistant should then load the mixed cement into the prepared crown or bridge.

3. The majority of composites today come in individual cartridges used with a syringe. The assistant assists with shade selection, loads the appropriate shade cartridge into the syringe, and passes it to the dentist. The assistant then passes shaping and contouring instruments, clear matrices, and the curing light if needed.

4. Bonding agents can be self-curing, light-cured, or dual-curing. Some are premixed in applicators, whereas others require mixing together two liquids. Each system typically includes three basic processes: etching, priming, and bonding. Follow the manufacturer's instructions. Assist with mixing and passing the components of the bonding system, keeping area clean and dry.

5. Glass ionomers are similar to some composites in their preparation and applications. They can be supplied as a powder and liquid that must be mixed before application or they are supplied in premixed application tubes or capsules. Follow the manufacturer's instructions for mixing and storage.

6. Intermediate restorative material (IRM) is available as premixed capsules that are triturated like amalgam or as liquid and powders that must be mixed before application. These materials do not last more than a year, but this is plenty of time for a provisional restoration.

7. Prepare varnishes, bases, and liners.

a. To prepare varnishes for use, open the bottle of varnish, dip the cotton pellet into the varnish, and transfer it to the dentist. Recap immediately to prevent thickening of varnish.

b. For bases, mix the cement materials until the consistency of putty and roll into two balls. Use a plastic filling instrument to pick up each ball and transfer it to the dentist.

c. For liners, dispense equal amounts of each paste onto opposite ends of a paper pad. Use a spatula to mix the pastes together. Transfer the liner to the dentist. Gather mixed pastes together onto end of spatula and pass to the dentist.

B. To prepare a provisional crown, prepare the liquid monomer and mix according to the manufacturer's directions. Load the resin into the prepared impression and transfer to the dentist.

III. Sedative and Palliative Materials

A. Periodontal surgical dressings can be formulated with or without zinc oxide eugenol. To mix, place equal lengths of the two pastes on a wax paper pad and mix with a wooden tongue depressor until uniform in color. When the paste loses its stickiness place it in a paper cup filled with room temperature water. Lubricate glove hands with water and form into strips and hand to the dentist.

B. Postextraction dressings can be periodontal dressings applied to the extraction sites to protect the sutures and can be either zinc oxide eugenol or eugenol free. They are mixed like periodontal dressings.

C. Sedative dressings are specifically formulated with zinc oxide eugenol, which has a sedative or palliative effect on the tissue. They are mixed the same way as other periodontal dressings.

IV. Prepare Other Dental Materials
   A. Tooth whitener should be prepared and applied according to the manufacturer's instructions. Some products can be applied with a special tray that is custom fitted to the patient's teeth. Others are brushed onto the tooth surface. Some materials are light-cured with a special light wand, whereas others must be continuously washed away and reapplied every 10 minutes during the procedure.
   B. Dental assistants use different endodontic materials to assist in root canal therapy. The filling material, called gutta-percha, is a rubber-like substance. Heat the filling material with a solvent before placing into the canal space. Gutta-percha is used in combination with an endodontic sealer. Sealers are available in either paste or powder and liquid form, which should be mixed according to manufacturer's instructions and transferred to the dentist.
   C. Apply etchants according to the manufacturer's instructions using the applicator or syringe.
   D. Apply sealants according to the manufacturer's directions. Cure the sealant if necessary, according to the manufacturer's instructions.

Review Questions

34. Which of the following cements have anticariogenic properties?
    A. Zinc polycarboxylate
    B. Zinc oxide eugenol
    C. Glass ionomer
    D. Zinc phosphate

35. Some materials give off heat when mixed. This is called a/an
    A. chemical reaction.
    B. exothermic reaction.
    C. thermal conductivity.
    D. thermal expansion.

36. A fluid's resistance to flow is called its
    A. flowability.
    B. viscosity.
    C. solubility.
    D. density.

37. A restoration that is created in the mouth is
    A. direct.
    B. indirect.
    C. preventive.
    D. chemical.

38. Dental bonding works by which of the following mechanisms?
    A. Creation of a smear layer to aid retention.
    B. Dissolution of the smear layer to aid retention.
    C. Creation of macromechanical retention.
    D. Creation of micromechanical retention.

39. Microleakage occurs when
    A. restorations are over-cured.
    B. the tooth is over-etched.
    C. contaminates are not removed.
    D. bonding material is excessive.

40. The organic matrix of composite resins is made up of
    A. BIS-GMA.
    B. glass.
    C. silica.
    D. quartz.

See p. 33 for the correct answers and rationales

Dental Materials and Laboratory Procedures

I.   Correctly Select Lab Materials and Mix and Handle Correctly
     A. Gypsum products are designated types I to V.
        1. Type I is an impression plaster and rarely used.
        2. Type II is a model plaster for preliminary impressions.
        3. Type III is a laboratory stone.
        4. Type IV is a die stone for bridges, crowns, and indirect restorations.
        5. Type V is a high-strength die stone.
        6. Orthodontic stone is used for orthodontic treatment.
        7. Measurements of water and powder must be exact. If too much water is used, the mix will be thin and runny. If too little water is used, the powder and water will not mix sufficiently or properly.
        8. Temperature of the water influences the setting time of the gypsum product: cool water—slows setting, warm water—speeds setting.
     B. Select and manipulate dental waxes.
        1. Use utility wax to extend the borders of an impression tray or cover metal orthodontic appliances.
        2. Use sticky wax to join objects together until they can be repaired or to form wax patterns.
        3. Use boxing wax to frame a preliminary impression.
        4. Use casting wax to create molds for indirect porcelain or metal restorations and also to fix bridges and metal portions of a partial denture.
        5. Use baseplate wax to create dentures.
        6. Use bite registration wax to make an imprint of the teeth.
     C. Store acrylic products and substitutes according to manufacturer's instructions.
     D. Correctly store all lab materials.
II. Performing Laboratory Procedures
     A. Fabricate, evaluate, trim, and finish diagnostic casts, including face bow mounting.
     B. Remove deposits and polish removable and fixed appliances and protheses.
     C. Remove deposits and polish complete and partial dentures.
     D. Fabricate mouth and athletic guards, custom impression and bleaching trays, and provisional prosthetics.

Review Questions

41. When stone is mixed with silica, it is referred to as
    A. a die stone.
    B. model plaster.
    C. porcelain.
    D. investment material.

42. How will the clinician know that it is safe to remove the poured model from the impression tray?
    A. The plaster/stone feels hard to the touch.
    B. The plaster/stone is no longer glossy.
    C. The plaster/stone is cool to the touch.
    D. The plaster/stone is warm to the touch.

43. Which of the following materials is most often used for veneers?
    A. Gold alloys
    B. Composites
    C. Porcelain
    D. Amalgams

See p. 33 for the correct answers and rationales

Educating and Assisting Patients with Oral Health

I. Patient Oral Health Education
    A. Plan and deliver dental health education information for the patient and community groups.
       1. Inform the patient of the importance of primary and permanent teeth in the relationship to supporting the jaw.
       2. Inform the patient of the causes of dental disease.
       3. Instruct the patient on the process of eruption and loss of teeth.
       4. Inform the patient of occlusal relationships, classifications, and their importance.
       5. Tell patients about saliva's role in oral health.
       6. Help patients choose the best restorative materials and procedures for their needs.
       7. Educate patients on how systemic health affects healing.
       8. Inform patient groups on how to adapt to their special needs
       9. Inform patients of the importance of their self-care and how to accomplish optimum oral health.
    B. Good communication is necessary for exchanging important information as well as building positive relationships with patients. Focus conversations on office procedures, policies, and patient care.
    C. Educate the patient on the advantages, disadvantages, delivery methods, and safe use of the different types of fluoride.
II. Instructions Before and After Treatment
    A. Deliver written and oral instructions to the patient before and after treatment including medication instructions.
    B. Provide written instructions to take home for patients to maintain and care for their dentures, including how to store and clean them. Also, advise patients not to attempt to adjust their dentures but, instead, to see their dentist with any problems.
III. Assisting Patients with Plaque Control
    A. Document the dentist's findings during clinical examinations. Record the findings and plans for treatment and follow-up care on specially designed forms that go in the patient's record.
    B. Educate patients on effective self-care oral health regimen. Especially as the number of dental products on the consumer market proliferates, make sure that patients are armed with solid information.
    C. Toothbrushes are available in many styles and shapes, but most dentists recommend soft bristles. Instruct patients on proper brushing technique.
       1. Tell patients to brush their teeth for 2 to 3 minutes, following the same pattern every time, twice a day.
       2. There are several techniques to guide patients in the right motions to both clean teeth and stimulate the gingiva, including Bass and modified Bass brushing technique, modified Stillman brushing technique, and the Charters brushing technique.
    D. Explain to patients the function of disclosing agents and how they operate. Then either apply the liquid disclosing agent or have the patient chew the tablet. Supply the patient with a hand-held mirror so he or she can inspect the results.

E. Help patients understand the wide selection of oral hygiene products available and what will work best for them.
1. Remind patients of the benefits of using floss and dental tape, both in caries prevention and gingival health.
2. Tell patients that oral irrigation is particularly helpful for them if they cannot or will not floss or if they have oral appliances that make adequate flossing difficult.
3. Instruct patients on interdental aids, such as interproximal brushes and dental stimulators, used to complement adequate brushing and flossing.
4. Explain to patients that mouth rinses are used to flush debris from the oral cavity, freshen the breath, and deliver fluoride.
F. Assess the patient's oral health regarding their ability to perform homecare procedures.
IV. Nutritional Education
A. Help patients understand how nutrition and lifestyle habits contribute to healthy teeth and gingiva. Proper nutrition is one of the most important ways to prevent dental caries. When educating patients about diet, consider several factors before giving recommendations: the patient's age, geographic background, medical conditions, and social and financial situation.
B. Sugar increases the risk of tooth decay. Rather than trying to eliminate sugar completely, encourage patients to decrease consumption of sugary foods and drinks. Patients can defend against the effects of sugar by brushing their teeth right after eating sweet treats. Although complex carbohydrates are converted to sugar in the body, they do not promote bacteria growth as quickly as simple carbohydrates. Encourage patients to stick to complex carbohydrates as much as possible, which are healthier in general.

Review Questions

44. Which of the following will occur as a result of ingesting too much fluoride?
A. Anodontia
B. Caries
C. Mottled enamel
D. Decalcification

45. Before topical fluoride is applied to a patient's teeth, the dental assistant should
A. recline the patient to a supine position.
B. have the patient rinse with mouthwash.
C. dry the teeth thoroughly.
D. use disclosing solution to look for plaque.

46. Toothbrushing alone has the ability to clean which of the following tooth surfaces?
A. Buccal
B. Occlusal pits and fissures
C. Lingual pits
D. Interproximal surfaces

47. Although sealants are most commonly placed on permanent molars, they may also be placed on deciduous teeth that
A. have deep pits and fissures.
B. have high caries activity.
C. are ready to exfoliate.
D. have shallow pits and fissures.

48. The main role of the dental assistant in preventive dentistry is
    A. dispensing fluoride rinses.
    B. taking radiographs.
    C. recording data.
    D. educating patients.

49. Which of the following microorganisms must be present in order for caries formation to begin?
    A. Staphylococci
    B. *Streptococcus mutans*
    C. Herpes zoster
    D. *Candida albicans*

See p. 33 for the correct answers and rationales

Medical and Dental Emergencies

I. Medical Emergencies
  A. The best way to prepare for, and hopefully prevent, a medical emergency is to be alert and gather as much information as possible about the patient.
     1. Patients who have AIDS should be questioned regarding their CD-4 helper T-cell count. If the count is below 200, their immune system is too weakened to withstand the stresses of dental treatment.
     2. Alcoholics frequently have advanced liver disease, compromising their blood clotting ability. The dental team should be prepared to deal with excessive bleeding problems.
     3. When obtaining a history from a patient, list drug allergies and repeat the information on each page of the record.
     4. Patients who have angina should be questioned about the frequency of their angina attacks, if they are well controlled, and when the last one occurred. If patients are experiencing frequent uncontrolled attacks, they should be referred to their physician. All patients with angina should have their nitroglycerin tablets with them and readily available during dental treatment.
     5. Arthritis symptoms may worsen throughout the day, so patients who have arthritis may prefer morning appointments. Be aware of the need for assistance getting in and out of the dental chair, comfort level in the chair, and ability to open the mouth and assume other positions as requested.
     6. When treating patients who have asthma, obtain information about triggers, frequency, and last asthma attack. If the asthma is poorly controlled, or stress induced, physician consultation is recommended. Asthma patients should always bring their inhalers with them to dental treatment and have them readily available for use.
     7. Depending on the type of blood dyscrasia, treatment modifications may be needed to prevent emergencies. Patients with low white blood cell counts are at risk for infection and poor healing, so elective treatment should be postponed until their white blood cell count improves. Patients with bleeding disorders need to have their clotting times evaluated and a physician's consult before any treatment that could cause bleeding. Patients who are anemic are at risk for hypoxia, and supplemental oxygen may be required
     8. The patient who is undergoing cancer treatment should always have a physician consult before dental treatment to avoid introducing infections due to their immunocompromised status. Cancer survivors may have residual oral problems such as osteoradionecrosis or salivary dysfunction. The mandible is a common site for cancer metastasis, so any oral problem should be have careful follow-up.
     9. Patients with heart disorders may need special care, including avoiding stress, keeping them in a semi-upright position, monitoring vital signs before and during treatment, and administering supplemental oxygen during treatment.
     10. Patients who have diabetes may have gingival irritation, alveolar bone loss, acetone breath, and delayed healing. Also, be sure to tell patients who have diabetes to eat normally before a dental appointment to prevent low blood sugar. Always have some sort of sugar source should a diabetic go into insulin shock (whereby they have insufficient glucose in their system).

11. Patients with chronic obstructive pulmonary disease may need to have the dental chair positioned more upright and have frequent drinks of water during treatment. Some patients' breathing may worsen throughout the day, so try to schedule morning appointments. Oxygen via cannula should be available, but dose delivered should never be over 2-3 L/min to avoid shutting down the hypoxic drive.

12. For a patient with epilepsy, ask if the patient is taking his or her medications, is eating regularly, well rested, or under stress. Also, ask if he or she has an aura that indicates a seizure, so the dental team can take appropriate measures.

13. Liver disease compromises clotting, so the patient should be carefully monitored for excess bleeding.

14. If a patient's blood pressure reading is too high, reschedule the patient—or even have them transported immediately to the hospital. To prevent orthostatic hypotension, raise the patient in the dental chair slowly and encourage them to remain reclined against the chair for a few minutes.

15. Patients with kidney or liver function problems may have problems with swelling, bleeding, or proper drug metabolism and excretion. Care should be exercised in prescribing medications and anesthesia administration to avoid toxicity.

16. Patients who have a compromised heart may need to take antibiotics prior to dental procedures to prevent bacteria from entering their bloodstream. Ensure that patients take medication before the appointment.

17. Patients with respiratory problems may need to be placed in a more upright position. A preprocedural rinse is especially important to avoid aspiration of harmful oral microorganisms into the lungs.

18. If there is damage to the heart valves due to rheumatic fever or congenital heart disease, the patient may need to receive prophylactic antibiotic premedication before dental treatment. A physician's consult is advised.

19. Patients with ulcers may experience internal bleeding and become severely anemic. Supplemental oxygen may be indicated.

20. For patients with venereal disease, if oral lesions exist, care must be taken not to spread them to other sites.

B. Understand how various classes and types of medications, patients may be taking, can affect bodily functions and how these effects might influence dental care, carefully documenting both prescription drugs and those purchased over the counter (OTC).

C. Be aware of the potential side effects, synergistic effects, and adverse effects of medications patients are taking that may interfere with the administration and effectiveness of drugs used during dental care. Careful monitoring is important. If a narcotic agent is given for sedation or pain relief, a narcotic antagonist (reverses the drug effect) should be available to prevent oversedation.

D. During a medical emergency, stay alert; quickly and correctly assess the situation.

1. The symptoms of an airway obstruction are usually immediate and obvious. Conscious patients who are choking frequently make the universal distress signal. Unconscious patients may quickly experience cardiac arrest.

2. Cardiovascular and cerebrovascular problems

    a. Symptoms of heart attacks vary among different people. Typically, the person experiences crushing or shooting chest pain or pressure, numbness in the left arm, dizziness, fainting (syncope), and heavy sweating. The person may also experience abdominal pain, back pain, and other non–chest-oriented symptoms.

    b. During a bout of angina, the patient experiences chest pains and may become dizzy or have trouble breathing. They may become pale and fearful. It is important to administer nitroglycerin sublingually immediately. If the patient does not respond after three doses, 5 minutes apart, they are experiencing a heart attack; emergency medical services (EMS) should be activated immediately.

    c. Symptoms of a stroke are an unsteady gait, confusion, a sudden and intense headache, along with vomiting, fainting and nausea, partial paralysis, vision disturbances, and a sudden loss of the ability to speak clearly. With a stroke, paralysis is on one side only, so that is an important diagnostic tool.

3. Problems related to diabetes or epilepsy

    a. If a diabetic patient is experiencing hyperglycemia, he or she may need to urinate excessively, become groggy and confused, and experience nausea. If a patient is experiencing hypoglycemia, he or she might become dizzy, have a pounding heartbeat, double vision, and fatigue, or may become unconscious.

    b. Patients with seizure disorders may experience an aura prior to a seizure.

4. Contact dermatitis is extremely rare, as are allergic reactions to local anesthetics. Patients may experience transient increase in heart rate due to the vasoconstrictor. Local anesthetic toxicity can occur if too much local anesthetic is administered, but it occurs as seizures, then loss of consciousness.

5. Respiratory problems
   a. When a patient hyperventilates, he or she may feel faint, numb, or groggy.
   b. Symptoms of an asthma attack range from mild wheezing to severe attacks.

6. Shock is a drastic drop in blood pressure that causes insufficient blood supply to the vital organs. The patient's blood pressure drops rapidly, the pulse becomes rapid, and collapse occurs quickly.

E. Respond appropriately to chairside emergencies.

1. Assist the dentist in the treatment of allergy attacks with antihistamines and epinephrine.

2. During a patient hemorrhage, apply local pressure and cold to diminish bleeding, place the patient in a supine position, and if bleeding does not abate, contact EMS.

3. Cardiovascular and cerebrovascular problems
   a. During a heart attack, if the patient is alert and awake, assist the dentist in the administration of oxygen along with nitroglycerin pills and baby aspirin. An unconscious patient may have gone into ventricular fibrillation and cardiac arrest, and requires cardiopulmonary resuscitation (CPR) and defibrillation with an automated external defibrillator (AED).
   b. Allow the patient to self-administer prescribed nitroglycerin.
   c. For strokes, place the patient in a reclining position on the affected side, contact EMS, and administer oxygen.

4. Emergencies related to metabolic and neurologic disease
   a. Insulin should never be administered by anyone except by physician order, so the dental assistant should activate EMS for emergency transport after being instructed by the dentist. The dental assistant can offer orange juice or a sugared drink upon instructions from the dentist.
   b. For seizures, remove everything from the patient's mouth, including tools and devices. Do not restrain the patient, but allow him or her to pass through the seizure episode. Protect the patient by moving furniture, equipment, etc., away from him or her.

5. Respiratory problems
   a. Assist patients who are having an asthma attack in using their inhaled bronchodilators.
   b. Treat choking by sitting the patient up and having them attempt to cough or spit the object out. If this is not successful, attempt the Heimlich maneuver. In unconscious patients, perform a finger-sweep in the patient's mouth and provide CPR as needed.

6. A patient in shock should be placed in a supine position. EMS should be activated immediately. Until the arrival of EMS, monitor vital signs and administer oxygen.

7. With transient unconsciousness, reposition the patient to a supine position and administer oxygen.

F. Every dental office should have an emergency kit stocked with basic medical supplies, as well as drugs that might be necessary in a medical emergency.

G. Emergency numbers should be posted next to every phone in the office, in an easy-to-locate spot.

II. Dental Emergencies

A. The most common dental emergency is syncope. Hypoglycemic episodes, angina, and asthma may be brought on by dental anxiety.

B. During a phone call with a distressed patient, only give advice under the direction of the dentist, or get the dentist on the phone.

Review Questions

50. Which of the following is a way to treat a patient having a hypoglycemic attack?
    A. Allow the patient to use a bronchodilator.
    B. Give the patient carbohydrates.
    C. Perform CPR on the patient.
    D. Remove everything from the patient's mouth.

51. If a patient has a grand mal seizure while in the office, the staff should
    A. stand back and let the seizure run its course.
    B. place the patient in an upright and seated position.
    C. clear away any hazards and call EMS.
    D. try to open the patient's airway.

52. Nitroglycerin is placed under the tongue of a patient who is experiencing
    A. heart failure.
    B. angina.
    C. a cerebrovascular accident.
    D. a severe allergic reaction.

53. In case of a medical emergency in the dental office
    A. all employees should be trained to render assistance.
    B. one person should be assigned to help the victim.
    C. the patient should rescheduled and sent home.
    D. a staff member should transport the patient to a hospital.

54. Treatment for a choking patient would begin when
    A. the patient becomes unconscious.
    B. the patient begins coughing vigorously.
    C. the patient's breathing and speech are impaired.
    D. the patient asks for assistance.

55. A patient who passes out immediately after dental treatment is most likely suffering from
    A. an allergic reaction.
    B. anesthetic overdose.
    C. syncope.
    D. hypoglycemia.

56. Symptoms of a patient suffering from a partially obstructed airway include
    A. loss of consciousness.
    B. excessive salivation.
    C. wheezing.
    D. respiratory distress.

57. A blood pressure reading of 140/90 indicates the patient has
    A. normal blood pressure.
    B. prehypertension.
    C. stage 1 hypertension.
    D. angina.

See p. 33 for the correct answers and rationales

Assisting in Dental Office Management

I. Maintain Adequate Supplies and Inventory Control
    A. Be sure that the cabinets are well stocked with the appropriate supplies needed in each treatment area. An efficient inventory control system includes a way to recognize when dental supplies are running low, a way to order them, and subsequently store them when they arrive. Inventory consists of expendable items that are consumed quickly and frequently reordered and nonexpendable items like machinery and equipment that is rarely replaced.
    B. Maintain accurate records of drugs prescribed or dispensed to patients. Order prescription pads and ensure that they are kept in a secure place; place controlled substances in locked cabinets to keep them secure.

II. Properly Maintain Equipment and Instruments

   A. Maintain the supply of instruments by making sure the office is fully equipped with the proper instruments in top working condition. Clean and sterilize dental instruments.

   B. Maintain sterility of disposable items and effectiveness of nitrous oxide and oxygen by proper care and storage.

   C. Maintain the cutting edge of the hand instruments by use of mechanical and manual methods.

III. Patient Management

   A. Establish good communication for exchanging important information as well as building positive relationships with patients, coworkers, and supervisors.

   B. After entering the reception area and identifying the patient by name, smile, greet the patient courteously while making eye contact, introduce yourself, and politely ask him or her to follow you back to the treatment area. When dismissing a patient, follow a series of steps that includes removing equipment from around the patient, updating the patient's record, and escorting the patient to the reception area.

   C. Dental appointments are scheduled in units of time in the appointment book—each procedure should be allotted enough units of time to enable its completion.

   D. On a patient's first visit to a dental practice, the patient is also entering into a financial arrangement with the business. With the patient's financial information in hand, treatment can be given or suggested. Dentists charge fees for their treatment commensurate with the type of treatment provided. If advised by the dentist, the dental assistant can provide information about treatment fees.

   E. For complicated, more expensive procedures that might require financing, patients may also have to give permission for the office to access their credit reports. This is an important document for dental offices that offer financing to patients, essentially loaning their patients money at an agreed-upon interest rate.

   F. Facilitate patient referrals under the dentist's instructions.

   G. Make sure you are trained to efficiently and effectively use the computers in the dental office.

IV. Legal Considerations for Dentistry

   A. A patient record is both a medical and a legal collection of documents and treatment tools.

      1. Legally, patients' medical histories are protected health information. During the course of taking a medical history, or using one in the office, the information should always remain confidential and be released only for purposes of treatment, payment, or oversight (governmental audits, accreditation, etc.).

      2. A patient record includes examination progress, test results, diagnoses, treatments, and legal forms, such as privacy and consent documents and registration forms.

      3. Dental practices are required to have a written privacy policy that is in compliance with the Health Insurance Portability and Accountability Act, or HIPAA. The law stipulates which kinds of information are considered privileged medical information and lays out the conditions under which sharing this information is allowed.

      4. Many different types of patient data are kept in the dental office.

         a. The dental history form is obtained from patients at the beginning of their treatment.

         b. A clinical examination form includes detailed information from the clinical examination, including charting, the patient's chief complaint, results from evaluations, and comments from the dentist.

         c. The medical history contains a record of the patient's past and present medical conditions.

         d. The consent form is a form given to new patients that obtain patient consent for dental exams and treatment.

         e. The privacy form is a signed acknowledgement that the patient received and understands the HIPAA privacy policy.

         f. Patient correspondence is any letters between the patient and the dental office.

         g. Radiographs and photographs

         h. Diagnostic or laboratory models

      5. File items are retained not only as hard (paper) copies, but also as digital files accessible via computer.

      6. Any letters between the patient and the dental office should be included in the patient record. This includes phone calls, emails, photos, or any other communication that might be pertinent to a patient's dental treatment.

   B. A dental practice is governed by a combination of federal, state, and local laws.

      1. Risk management includes professional and office practices designed to reduce the risk of injury to patients and employees—and therefore the risk of lawsuit. It starts with personal behavior and responsibility, such as following professional codes and standards, documenting patient treatments and consent, maintaining professional competence, and following the four Cs of malpractice prevention.

2. When a dentist explains a procedure to a patient and the patient signs an agreement indicating that he or she understands the procedure, is aware of possible complications, and agrees that the procedure should be done, this is a written agreement between the dentist as the service provider and the patient as the recipient of the service. It is called informed consent. When a patient comes in and allows the dentist to conduct an examination, this implies treatment is wanted. No written contract is needed and this is implied consent.

3. As a dental assistant, you owe a duty of care to the dentist to make sure that properly signed and dated consent forms are in the patient's chart before the treatment or procedure is performed.

4. HIPAA ensures the privacy and confidentiality of patient healthcare information. HIPAA requirements apply to all direct and indirect healthcare providers.

5. Within a dental practice, the dentist is viewed as ultimately responsible for the work of all others in the practice. It can be an important legal protection for you if you are ever accused of a tort. This legal principle applies when the actions you take are within your scope of practice, so you should always be on guard against acting outside your scope of practice.

6. The state dental practice act spells out requirements dental assistants, dentists, and dental hygienists need to meet in order to obtain and maintain licenses or registration within that state. The act sets up requirements for state board examinations and for continuing education. Each state's act also explains the conditions under which a license can be renewed, suspended, or revoked.

7. If a patient refuses an examination, treatment, or test, document the refusal in the chart. If possible, ask the patient to sign a statement indicating that he or she is refusing treatment and keep that statement in the chart.

8. All dental assistants must be thoroughly acquainted with the regulatory and professional bodies of the Centers for Disease Control and Prevention and Occupational Safety and Health Administration. Offices should have an inspection and enforcement mechanism in place to make sure they are compliant.

Review Questions

58. Communication through body language is what kind of communication?
    A. Verbal
    B. Nonverbal
    C. Active listening
    D. Passive listening

59. Which of the following is the next logical step after presentation of the patient's treatment plan?
    A. Treatment should start immediately without regard to financial arrangements.
    B. Treatment should be delayed until all payments can be made.
    C. The dentist or other dental team member discusses estimated fees and makes financial arrangements.
    D. The dentist or other dental team member submits estimated fees to the insurance company.

60. The Health Insurance Portability and Accountability Act stipulates that protected health information can be released to which of the following persons?
    A. Patient's spouse
    B. Patient's brother
    C. Patient's children
    D. Patient only

61. A dentist who refuses to treat a patient in need of dental care, without giving adequate notice to the patient, has committed which of the following?
    A. Abandonment
    B. A felony
    C. Fraud
    D. Malpractice

See p. 33 for the correct answers and rationales

ANSWERS AND RATIONALES:
General Chairside

Collecting and Recording Clinical Data

1. Using the universal numbering system, the permanent maxillary right second molar is tooth number

    A. 2. In the universal numbering system, the permanent teeth are numbered 1–32, beginning with the maxillary right third molar (tooth number 1). The permanent maxillary right second molar is tooth number 2.

2. A small, rounded extension of bone covered with soft tissue located posterior to the last maxillary molar is the

    C. maxillary tuberosity. The maxillary tuberosity is located behind the last maxillary molar.

3. Which of the following best describes the palantine rugae?

    B. Horizontally raised folds of hard tissue behind the incisive papilla on the hard palate. The palantine rugae are raised fold-like ridges of keratinized tissue behind the incisive papilla. They are as distinctive as fingerprints.

4. To identify Stensen's papilla, look for a

    A. small raised flap of soft tissue on the buccal mucosa opposite the maxillary second molar. Stensen's papilla, often marked with small red dot, is a small raised flap of soft tissue on the buccal mucosa just opposite the maxillary first molar.

5. Which of the following nerves provides sensory innervation for the teeth and mouth?

    C. Trigeminal. In addition to the teeth and mouth, the trigeminal nerve also provides sensory innervation for the scalp and face.

6. Which of the following major salivary glands is located on the side of the face, behind the ramus, below and in front of the ear?

    B. Parotid. The parotid gland is the largest of the salivary glands.

General Dentistry Chairside Procedures

7. In rubber dam placement, the purpose of inverting the dam is to

    D. prevent saliva leakage. Inverting the dam creates a seal, which helps to prevent the leakage of saliva.

8. Which of the following instruments is likely to be included in a basic tray setup?

   B. Mouth mirror. Basic instruments are typically included in every tray setup and include a mouth mirror, explorer, cotton pliers, and periodontal probe.

9. A carious lesion in a pit or fissure would be classified as:

   A. Class I caries: a lesion located in a pit or fissure of a tooth. Class I caries are located on pits and fissures of the teeth in both anterior and posterior areas.

10. Which of the following is an example of biological pulpal stimuli?

    D. Bacteria from saliva coming into contact with pulpal tissues. Biological stimuli occur as a result of bacteria from saliva coming into contact with pulpal tissues.

11. What does an etchant remove in preparation for dental bonding?

    C. Smear layer. Bonding to the dentin first requires removal of the smear layer, which is a thin film of fluids and particles that forms over the dentin when a cavity is prepared.

12. Which of the following procedures uses enamel bonding?

    A. Sealant. Sealants are retained by the micromechanical bonds created after enamel etching.

13. Which instrument is used first during an amalgam restoration?

    A. Excavator. During an amalgam procedure, the excavator is used to remove any soft carious tissue from the tooth. After the amalgam is placed into the prep with the condenser, the cleoid-discoid carves the anatomy back into the amalgam of the occlusal surface of the tooth. Finally, a burnisher ward completes the anatomy and smooths it out.

14. Which one of the following tests provides a definitive diagnosis of oral cancer?

    D. Performing a biopsy. The only certain method of diagnosis for cancer is histological testing, or biopsy.

15. Which of the following may help prevent a patient from gagging during an alginate impression?

    B. Using warm water to mix the alginate. Using warm water to mix the alginate aids in shortening the length of the procedure for the patient by shortening the time that the impression material and tray must be in the patient's mouth.

16. The curing time of composite restorations depends on the

    A. shade of the restorative material. The darker the shade of the composite material, the longer the curing time required.

17. Which of the following must be done first when preparing a tooth for provisional coverage?

    C. Placement of the post and core. A preliminary impression must be taken before the tooth is prepared to obtain a reproduction of the tooth and surrounding tissues in order to fabricate a custom provisional.

18. When assisting during final impressions in a crown and bridge preparation, which elastomeric impression material is applied first to the teeth?

    A. Light-bodied. The light-bodied material is used first as it has the ability to flow into and around the details of the prepared teeth.

19. What is the operating zone for an assistant who is assisting a right-handed operator?

    B. 2 o'clock to 4 o'clock. If we look at the work area as a clock, the assistant's zone is from 2 to 4 o'clock.

20. Which part of an anesthetic syringe locks into the rubber stopper so that the stopper can be retracted by pulling back on the piston rod?

    D. Harpoon. This hook is at the end of the piston and locks into the rubber stopper of the cartridge, enabling the stopper to be retracted when the dentist pulls back on the thumb ring.

21. During a class II amalgam procedure, when is the wedge removed?

    A. Before the matrix band and holder are removed. To safeguard the integrity of the newly placed amalgam restoration, the wedge is removed before removing the matrix band. If the matrix band is removed before the wedge is removed, the new restoration is more likely to fracture.

22. When preparing a Tofflemire matrix band and retainer, the inner nut on the retainer is used to

    C. adjust the size of the matrix band loop. After the band has been bent into shape, it is inserted into the diagonal slots on the retainer and positioned with the guide channels. Then it is screwed into place with the spindle pin. The size of the loop can be adjusted using the inner knob on the retainer.

23. Using the clock concept, the zone located between 4 o'clock and 7 o'clock when working with a right-handed operator is the

    D. transfer zone. When working with a right-handed operator, the transfer zone is under patient's chin and above the patient's chest.

24. When an instrument is held in the palm of the hand with all four fingers surrounding the instrument and the thumb supporting the instrument, which grasp is being used?

    D. Palm-thumb. The palm-thumb grasp is used with straight-line instruments where both precision and strength are necessary, such as chisels and hoes.

25. When passing an instrument that will be used on tooth number 17, the working end should be in what position?

    B. Downward toward the mandibular teeth. When transferring an instrument to be used on tooth number 17, the working end should be pointing downward for the mandibular area. When working in the maxillary region, the position of use for the instrument being transferred is upward toward the maxillary teeth.

26. Which of the following medications could increase the patient's blood pressure and heart rate?

    C. Over-the-counter cold medication. Although all of the medications can have an effect on dental treatment, over-the-counter cold medications mimic the sympathetic nervous system, increasing both heard rate (pulse) and blood pressure. Aspirin and warfarin could cause increased bleeding and nitroglycerin is prescribed for patients with angina pectoris, who are at risk for heart attacks.

27. In the United States, nitrous oxide tanks are color-coded

   C. blue. In the United States, nitrous oxide tanks are color-coded blue and oxygen tanks are color-coded green to prevent accidental mix-ups.

28. The drug of choice for dental and outpatient inflammatory pain is

   D. ibuprofen. Ibuprofen is a member of the nonsteroidal anti-inflammatory drug group and is the drug of choice because of its effectiveness in reducing pain and inflammation related to dental treatment.

29. Which drug would be contraindicated in patients with peptic ulcers?

   A. Aspirin. Aspirin causes gastrointestinal upset and even bleeding in some patients. Patients with peptic ulcers should never be given aspirin which could make the ulcer worse.

30. Nitrous oxide/oxygen inhalation is indicated for which of the following conditions?

   B. Dental anxiety. The anxious patient will benefit from the relaxing and analgesic effects of nitrous oxide/oxygen inhalation sedation. The other conditions would interfere with adequate respiration and would not allow the full effect of nitrous oxide.

31. Codeine is classified at what level of abuse and addiction potential?

   C. Schedule III. The Drug Enforcement Administration classifies codeine as a schedule III drug, which means it has a moderate potential for abuse and addiction and is a controlled substance.

32. Why would an oral surgeon administer diazepam (Valium) to a patient before extraction of a molar?

   B. To relieve anxiety. Diazepam (Valium) is of the benzodiazepine class of medications that is given to reduce anxiety. It is often used preoperatively for sedation.

33. What is the most commonly used formulation of topical anesthetic?

   D. 20% benzocaine. Twenty percent benzocaine is the most commonly used formulation of topical anesthetic used in dentistry today.

Preparing and Working with Chairside Materials

34. Which of the following cements have anticariogenic properties?

   C. Glass ionomer. Of the cements listed, glass ionomer cement has the unique ability to release fluoride after setting. Because of this, glass ionomer cements are useful in inhibiting decay.

35. Some materials give off heat when mixed. This is called a/an

   C. thermal conductivity. An exothermic reaction occurs when heat is given off as the result of a chemical reaction.

36. A fluid's resistance to flow is called its

   B. viscosity. The way a material flows is its viscosity. An example of a material with a high viscosity is cold maple syrup, which does not flow very easily. Warm maple syrup, however, has a lower viscosity and flows more easily.

37. A restoration that is created in the mouth is

   A. direct. A direct restoration is applied to the tooth/teeth while the restorative material is still pliable and can be easily adapted.

38. Dental bonding works by which of the following mechanisms?

   D. Creation of micromechanical retention. Bonding systems work by etching surfaces, creating microscopic areas that the bonding agent can flow into, and improve retention of the restorative material.

39. Microleakage occurs when

   C. contaminates are not removed. Contaminants can contribute to microleakage when they are not properly removed before and during the bonding process.

40. The organic matrix of composite resins is made up of

   A. BIS-GMA. The most commonly used resin for the matrix of composites is BIS-GMA, or dimethacrylate

Dental Materials and Laboratory Procedures

41. When stone is mixed with silica, it is referred to as

   D. investment material. When stone is mixed with silica, it forms dental investment, a material able to withstand the high heat and stress produced when molten metal is forced into molds to form indirect restorations.

42. How will the clinician know that it is safe to remove the poured model from the impression tray?

   C. The plaster/stone is cool to the touch. Gypsum products such as plaster and stone are exothermic (release heat) while the setting is occurring. The model will lose its glossy appearance at the initial set, but the reaction is not complete, and removing the model from the tray at this point can result in breakage. Once heat is no longer produced, and the model feels cool to the touch, it is safe to remove the model from the impression tray.

43. Which of the following materials is most often used for veneers?

   C. Porcelain. Although porcelain is effective in making teeth appear healthier and more natural looking, as a material, it is not very strong and does not resist fracturing as well as other materials. This is why porcelain is generally used in making veneers, not inlays, onlays, or crowns.

General Chairside

Educating and Assisting Patients with Oral Health

44. Which of the following will occur as a result of ingesting too much fluoride?

C. Mottled enamel. Dental fluorosis, also referred to as mottling or mottled enamel, is caused by ingesting too much fluoride during the development and mineralization of the teeth.

45. Before topical fluoride is applied to a patient's teeth, the dental assistant should

C. dry the teeth thoroughly. Teeth should be thoroughly dried using the air-water syringe and/or a gauze sponge to remove saliva and any remaining toothpaste prior to applying a topical fluoride treatment.

46. Toothbrushing alone has the ability to clean which of the following tooth surfaces?

A. Buccal. Tooth brushing alone cleans the buccal and lingual tooth surfaces. Deep occlusal fissures, pits, fossa, as well as lingual pits cannot be adequately cleaned by tooth brushing alone. Tooth brushing also cannot interproximal and subgingival areas.

47. Although sealants are most commonly placed on permanent molars, they may also be placed on deciduous teeth that

A. have deep pits and fissures. To reduce the risk of decay, pit and fissure sealants are commonly used on deciduous molars where deep occlusal grooves, pits, and fissures are present.

48. The main role of the dental assistant in preventive dentistry is

D. educating patients. Patients need to be thoroughly educated on how to care for their mouth at home in order for what is done at the dental office to be successful.

49. Which of the following microorganisms must be present in order for caries formation to begin?

B. *Streptococcus mutans*. Dental caries is a transmittable bacterial infection that is caused by the mutans streptococcus or the lactobacilli.

Medical and Dental Emergencies

50. Which of the following is a way to treat a patient having a hypoglycemic attack?

B. Give the patient carbohydrates. Giving the patient a glucose supplement will help to raise the patient's blood sugar.

51. If a patient has a grand mal seizure while in the office, the staff should

C. clear away any hazards and call EMS. A patient having a seizure should be allowed to lie on the floor with hazards moved away to prevent serious injury. As with any emergency, EMS should be activated so that the patient can receive optimum emergency care.

52. Nitroglycerin is placed under the tongue of a patient who is experiencing

    B. angina. The drug of choice for a patient experiencing chest pain due to angina pectoris is nitroglycerine. It is administered by placing a tablet sublingually.

53. In case of a medical emergency in the dental office

    A. all employees should be trained to render assistance. All staff members should be trained in basic first aid and CPR. Periodic mock drills of different emergencies should be run in order for staff to know what their responsibility is in case an emergency should occur. Emergency phone numbers should be posted at every phone in the office.

54. Treatment for a choking patient would begin when

    C. the patient's breathing and speech are impaired. If a patient's airway becomes blocked and he or she can no longer speak, then treatment should begin by performing abdominal thrusts to relieve the obstruction. As long as the patient is talking, coughing, and breathing then they should be allowed to attempt to clear the obstruction on their own.

55. A patient who passes out immediately after dental treatment is most likely suffering from

    C. syncope. Syncope, or fainting, often occurs right after a dental appointment if the patient has been supine for a long period of time and then exits the dental chair quickly.

56. Symptoms of a patient suffering from a partially obstructed airway include

    C. wheezing. Symptoms of a patient suffering from a partially obstructed airway include wheezing. A patient suffering from a completely obstructed airway would show signs of respiratory distress and possible loss of consciousness.

57. A blood pressure reading of 140/90 indicates the patient has

    C. stage 1 hypertension. A blood pressure reading of 140/90 indicates the patient has stage 1 hypertension. A normal blood pressure reading is 120/80.

Assisting in Dental Office Management

58. Communication through body language is what kind of communication?

    B. Nonverbal. Communication without words or language, including body gestures, facial expressions, and eye contact.

59. Which of the following is the next logical step after presentation of the patient's treatment plan?

    C. The dentist or other dental team member discusses estimated fees and makes financial arrangements. The treatment plan is a structured presentation of the patient's needs and the dentist or other dental team member should help the patient understand treatment needs and make financial arrangements. Once the patient has been informed, a pretreatment estimate can be sent to the insurance company.

60. HIPAA stipulates that protected health information can be released to which of the following persons?

   D. Patient only. HIPAA requires that only the patient's signed release of information allows others to view the patient's protected health information.

61. A dentist who refuses to treat a patient in need of dental care, without giving adequate notice to the patient, has committed which of the following?

   A. Abandonment. By law, a dentist must give a patient adequate notice prior to refusal to treat.

RADIATION HEALTH AND SAFETY (RHS)

Expose and Evaluate

I. Choice of Technique

    A. Understand the use and purpose of both intraoral and extraoral radiographs.

        1. A periapical radiograph includes an image of the whole tooth, from its occlusal surface or incisal edge to the apices and surrounding structures. It is used to diagnose conditions involving tooth formation and eruption.

        2. A bitewing exposure shows the crowns and alveolar bones of the mandibular and maxillary arch on one exposure. It is used to detect dental caries in posterior teeth and alveolar bone crests between teeth.

        3. Occlusal exposures visualize large areas of the upper and lower jaws and can locate extra, unerupted or impacted teeth, foreign bodies, salivary stones, lesions, or fractures.

        4. Panoramic radiography produces a large image of the maxilla and mandible on a single piece of film. It is used for lateral jaw, skull, and temporomandibular radiographs.

        5. Encephalometric and other extraoral views

            a. Skull radiographs visualize larger areas of the skull, jaws, and bones of the face and sometimes require a cephalostat to position the head. These radiographs are used by oral surgeons and orthodontics for fractures and development of the jaw.

            b. Lateral jaw radiographs visualize the posterior region of the mandible. They are used for impacted molars, fractures, and large areas of pathological concern.

            c. Temporomandibular joint (TMJ) radiographs visualize the mandibular condyle, the glenoid fossa, and the articular eminence. They are used to evaluate TMJ as well as diagnose fractures, tumors, and pathologies.

    B. Select appropriate radiographic film to examine conditions, teeth, and landmarks of patients.

        1. Bitewing radiographs most commonly detect dental caries in posterior teeth and alveolar bone crests between teeth.

        2. Temporomandibular joint (TMJ) radiographs evaluate TMJ.

        3. A full-mouth radiographic survey evaluates periodontal disease.

        4. Apical pathology includes abscesses, granuloma, and cysts.

        5. Waters projections visualize the maxillary sinus area.

        6. The occlusal technique reveals supernumerary teeth and other anomalies.

        7. For edentulous patients, perform the occlusal, periapical, and panoramic radiographs and use either the bisecting or the parallel technique.

        8. The occlusal technique locates unerupted or impacted teeth.

        9. Periapical, bitewings, and panoramic radiographs can be used for dental implants.

II. Radiographic Equipment

    A. Accessories for radiographic techniques

        1. Use film holders, such as bite blocks, during parallel radiography and in the bisecting technique to hold the film still in the patient's mouth.

        2. Cotton rolls help position and handle films.

        3. The film cassette holds the screen film and the two intensifying screens in close contact and protects the screen film from white light.

        4. Intensifying screens minimize radiation exposure.

        5. A bitewing tab is a paper tab that extends from the film, which patients clamp between their teeth.

        6. A lead apron is a protective device that shields patients from excess radiation exposure.

        7. A thyroid collar is a protective device worn by patients to protect the thyroid gland in the neck.

    B. Film speed has a letter classification system. A is the slowest film, whereas F is the fastest film. The American Dental Association and the American Academy of Oral and Maxillofacial Radiology recommend that only the E-speed or F-speed films be used. Currently, no film speed less than D-speed is used.

    C. Like any kind of film, store dental films carefully to prevent early exposure or film degradation.
        1. Protect dental film from stray radiation, moisture, temperature extremes, chemicals, and light.
        2. Ideal temperatures for dental film storage range between 50° and 72° F, with a relative humidity from 30% to 50%. Do not refrigerate dental film because of the risk of condensation and water damage.
        3. Store newer boxes toward the back, so older boxes with a more recent expiration date are used first.

III. Infection Control Techniques and Barriers
    A. The Centers for Disease Control and Prevention's (CDC) guidelines cover using barrier techniques and protective clothing, using heat-tolerant or disposable film-holding devices, cleaning and sterilizing film holders between patients, transporting and handling exposed film packets in a manner that reduces risk of infection, and cleaning and sterilizing digital sensors and other equipment.

IV. Patient Management Techniques During Radiographic Procedures
    A. Some patients may be worried about intraoral radiography because of the strange equipment, X-rays, or even holding film in their mouths. Help these patients by calmly and patiently explaining the procedure, as well as its benefits, so patients know what to expect.
    B. Use different techniques to manage patients while exposing radiographs.
        1. Some patients are unable to suppress their gag reflex during radiography. To help the patient, try distracting them, working quickly, using an anesthetic mouth rinse, and asking the patient to breathe through his or her mouth.
        2. Some patients have special needs or require a specialized approach.
            a. For children, make allowances the smaller oral cavity size. Pediatric patients also require less kilovoltage, milliamperage, and exposure time.
            b. When dealing with a development disability, work within the patient's limitations. Some patients may be unable to hold film holders in their mouths or they may experience involuntary movement that causes errors during exposure.
            c. In a patient with visual disabilities, communicate with clear verbal instructions and refrain from gesturing at other people in the room silently.
            d. With hearing-impaired people, it depends on the patient's preferred form of communication. Some people will prefer to read lips. In other cases, written instructions will work and, in still other cases, an interpreter or caregiver can serve as a go-between, using sign language.
            e. Patients with mobility impairments include those who are in wheelchairs; those who may have lost the use of their legs, arms, or both; or those who are unable to raise or lower themselves into the dental chair. If it is possible, transfer a patient into the dental chair. If not, radiographs can be taken with a patient still seated in a wheelchair.

V. Techniques for Exposing Dental Films
    A. Understand the definitions of exposure concepts.
        1. Film speed is a measure of the film's sensitivity to radiation.
        2. Kilovolt (kV) is a unit of electrical potential, equal to 103 volts; in dental radiography, it is a measure of the power of the dental X-ray unit.
        3. Milliampere (mA) is one thousandth of an amp; in dental radiography, it is a measure of how many electrons are contained in an X-ray.
        4. Collimator is a lead-based safety device in the X-ray tubehead that focuses and targets the X-ray beam as it emerges from the X-ray tube.
        5. Filtration removes the long wavelength, poorly penetrating radiation that would be absorbed by the patient's skin.
        6. Density is the overall darkness of the film and needs to be appropriate for diagnostic quality: Dark enough to detect the images of interest, but not too dark to obscure them. Density can be controlled by adjusting exposure time, peak kV (kVp), or mA.
        7. A latent image is a radiographic image stored on dental film after exposure but before processing.
    B. Intraoral exposures
        1. Understand factors that affect the quality of exposure.
            a. A higher mA equals increased density; a lower mA equals decreased density.
            b. A higher kVp means increased density, long-scale contrast, and low contrast; a lower kVp means decreased density, short-scale contrast, and high contrast.
            c. Vertical angulation describes the orientation of the positron indicating device (PID) in a vertical plane around the patient's head. Positive vertical angulation means the PID is pointing toward the floor. Negative vertical angulation means the PID is pointing toward the ceiling. Horizontal

angulation describes the orientation of the PID in a horizontal plane around the patient's head. The central X-ray beam should be aimed directly through the spaces between the patient's teeth.

   d. In foreshortening, the PID is not angled at a steep enough angle to capture an accurate image of the structure of interest.

   e. Common placement errors are absence of apical structures, absence of crown structure, tilted image or dropped film corner, and angulation problems.

   f. Underexposure results in a light image and can be caused by inadequate exposure time. Overexposure results in a dark image and can be caused by excessive exposure time.

2. Two basic techniques used to obtain exposure types are parallel and bisecting.

   a. The parallel technique, where the film is held parallel to the long axis of the tooth, yields superior radiographs with less exposure. A disadvantage is that patients may experience discomfort with the bite blocks.

   b. In the bisecting technique, the film is placed against the tooth at an angle. It is valuable when the parallel technique is not an option, but there is some distortion of the resulting image. Also, foreshortening and elongation are more common and there is greater radiation exposure.

3. Dental film packets have a waterproof outer package to protect the film, black paper on either side of the film itself, the radiograph film, and a lead foil backing to reduce the amount of scatter radiation that would expose the patient to unnecessary radiation and fog the film.

C. Obtain extraoral radiographs by placing the film outside the patient's mouth.

1. Intensifying screens minimize radiation exposure. They convert X-ray energy into visible light, which then exposes the screen film. Each film cassette contains two intensifying screens, one in front of and one behind the film.

2. Use appropriate techniques for exposing radiographs.

   a. Patient position is critical in panoramic radiography to make sure the dental arches are positioned in the focal trough. The following conditions are required: the midsagittal plane should be perpendicular to the floor, the ala-tragus line should be inclined toward the floor about 5 degrees, and the Frankfort plane should be parallel to the floor.

   b. Cephalometric radiography

      1. Lateral skull projections require use of film positioned in a cassette directly over the patient's shoulder. Position the patient's head between the cassette film with the intensifying screens and the X-ray tubehead. Place the cassette parallel to the midsagittal plane of the skull. Direct the central X-ray beam at the acoustic meatus with a fixed vertical angulation of zero degrees.

      2. The posteroanterior cephalometric, or PA projection, is the companion exposure to the lateral skull radiography. PA projections require the use of the cephalostat to position the head relative to the X-ray beam and the film. Film is used with intensifying screens. The film cassette is positioned in front of the patient, so he or she is looking into the film, with the nose and forehead touching the cassette. Vertical angulation is zero degrees, and the central X-ray beam is directed at the external occipital protuberance (the large bump near the base of the skull).

VI. Digital Radiography

A. Digital radiography uses electronic sensors or phosphor plates to store X-ray energy and convert it to digital images. It requires less radiation and the images are immediately available.

VII. Evaluating Dental Radiographs

A. Make sure the image captures the teeth and bone structures, showing all the relevant areas. It should be a clear image with minimal distortion or none at all. Images should not be elongated, foreshortened, magnified, or distorted in any way. There should be a clear contrast on the film between light and dark areas.

B. Errors resulting from exposure problems

1. Elongation results from insufficient angulation.

2. Foreshortening results from excessive vertical angulation.

3. Incorrect horizontal angulation results in overlapping images from adjacent teeth, obscuring the interproximal contact areas.

4. Cone cuts appear as clear areas on the film. This happens when the PID is aligned incorrectly and the central X-ray beam does not expose the entire surface of the film. Cone cuts also occur with the use of rectangular PIDs, which reduce the amount of radiation exposure by more tightly focusing the central X-ray beam, but require additional care in placement.

5. Underexposure results in a light image. Underexposure can be caused by inadequate exposure time, kilovoltage, or milliamperage, or by too much distance between the film and the PID.

6. Overexposure results in a dark image. This can be caused by excessive exposure time, kilovoltage, or milliamperage.

7. If the film is bent excessively during exposure, the teeth will appear rounded or stretched. This typically occurs when the curvature of the palate is excessive and pressure from the patient's mouth is bending the film. To prevent this, cotton rolls can be used with the parallel technique to release pressure on the film. Film-holding devices are also helpful in preventing this.

8. A herringbone pattern across the surface of the radiograph means that the film was reversed in the patient's mouth during exposure. The herringbone pattern is created by the embossed lead foil backing on the film. These films are also significantly underexposed. To correct this, make sure that the film is facing the correct way, with the tube side toward the teeth and X-ray beam.

9. Cone cuts appear as clear areas on the film.

10. Patient movement during exposure will result in blurry radiographs. To prevent this, the patient should be stabilized in a comfortable position, with his or her head firmly supported, before exposure.

11. Superimposed image

12. A double image is the result of accidentally exposing the same film twice. To prevent this, make sure exposed film is immediately placed in the proper spot.

13. After each exposure, the film should be removed carefully from the patient's oral cavity. Any saliva should be removed immediately by gently swiping the film with a disinfectant premoistened paper towel.

14. Placement errors are the most common problem with radiographs.
    a. With an absence of apical structure, the film packet was not placed either high enough or low enough during exposure. To correct this, make sure that no more than 2 mm of film extends beyond the occlusal/incisal edge of the tooth.
    b. With an absence of crown structure, the film was placed either not low enough or high enough during exposure. A lip of film measuring 2 mm should extend beyond the occlusal/incisal edge of the tooth to correctly expose the crown. The use of film holders and the correct size film can prevent this.
    c. A tilted image or dropped film corner results in a radiograph with a tilted occlusal plane. It is caused when the film edge is not placed parallel to the occlusal/incisal edge of the tooth. This most often occurs when an inferior or broken film holder is used. Also, the finger-holding technique results in tipped films. To fix, use a proper film holder.
    d. Angulation problems describe the position of the PID along the horizontal and vertical planes around the patient's head. Some common problems result from incorrect angulation. Overlapping contacts, which occur when the X-ray beam is not directed straight through the contact areas of the teeth, is an error in horizontal angulation. In foreshortened images, the teeth appear short, with rounded roots; this is caused by excessive vertical angulation in the bisecting technique. With elongated images, the teeth appear stretched; this is caused by insufficient vertical angulation in the bisecting technique.

C. Identify and correct common errors that take place during panoramic radiography.
    1. In positioning, if the Frankfort plane is not parallel to the floor, blurry regions, distortions, or other structures superimposed over the radiograph can result. If the midsagittal plane is misaligned, the teeth closest to the film appear smaller, whereas the teeth farthest from the film appear magnified. If the teeth are positioned either too far forward or too far back from the focal trough, the result is a blurred image. If the patient is positioned too far forward (anterior), the anterior teeth appear too thin, and if the patient is positioned too far back (posterior), the anterior teeth appear overlarge, or fat. If the patient's lips or tongue are in improper positions, radiolucent shadows will obscure parts of the image. The lips should be firmly enclosed around the bite block and the tongue should be positioned firmly against the roof of the mouth.
    2. Film cassette errors occur when the film is not matched to the proper color intensifying screens, oriented correctly in the cassette, and is not light-safe, resulting in accidental partial exposure.
    3. Exposure and processing errors can occur if the proper settings, including kV and mA, are not used. Larger patients with denser tissues will require higher kV.
    4. Patient cooperation errors occur when the patient does not hold still or holds their lips and tongue in the correct position. Make sure patients understand that there are moving components to a panoramic X-ray unit and that these components will be circling their head during exposure.

Review Questions

1. What characteristic will a radiograph exhibit if the film was placed backward in the mouth?
     A. Blurred image
     B. Clear film
     C. Herringbone effect
     D. Dark film

2. Elongation on a dental radiograph is caused by
     A. too much horizontal angle.
     B. too little horizontal angle.
     C. too much vertical angle.
     D. too little vertical angle.

3. When taking a radiograph of a 6-year-old patient, which of the following adjustments is made for the child's size?
     A. Higher kilovoltage
     B. Lower kilovoltage
     C. Shorter exposure time
     D. Longer exposure time

4. Cone cutting results when the central ray
     A. is not aimed at the center of the film.
     B. is aimed directly at the center of the film.
     C. has too much horizontal angulation.
     D. has too little vertical angulation.

5. If the distance between the tooth and the X-ray beam is decreased, the image will have
     A. decreased magnification.
     B. increased magnification.
     C. long-scale contrast.
     D. short-scale contrast.

6. Penumbra is the
     A. magnification of an object.
     B. negatively charged ion.
     C. distortion of the image.
     D. diffuse outline of the image.

7. Which of the following positioning errors results in an overlapped image?
     A. Incorrect vertical angulation
     B. Tubehead movement
     C. Incorrect horizontal angulation
     D. Patient movement

8. When using an aiming ring to align the PID, the rim on the open end of the tube should be
     A. parallel to the ring.
     B. perpendicular to the ring.
     C. positively angled.
     D. negatively angled.

9. Overlapping the contact areas on a bitewing radiograph is an indication that the
    A. horizontal angulation is off.
    B. vertical angulation is off.
    C. negative angulation is off.
    D. positive angulation is off.

10. Filters are used in the X-ray tubehead to reduce
    A. image density.
    B. exposure time.
    C. the size of the beam.
    D. the patient radiation dose.

11. How should film be repositioned when the third molar is not showing up on a radiograph of the mandibular molar area?
    A. Lower the film
    B. Raise the film
    C. Move the film forward in the mouth
    D. Move the film farther back in the mouth

12. The distal surface of the canine should be observed in which of the following radiograph exposures?
    A. Molar bitewing
    B. Premolar bitewing
    C. Lateral incisor periapical
    D. Central incisor periapical

13. Which of the following anatomical landmarks is not visible in the mandibular molar exposure?
    A. External oblique ridge
    B. Mental foramen
    C. Mandibular canal
    D. Mylohyoid ridge

14. The horizontal line from the top of the ear through the corner of the eye that is used for positioning a patient for a panoramic film is the
    A. ala-tragus line.
    B. midsagittal plane.
    C. Frankfort plane.
    D. transcranial line.

15. Occlusal radiographs are used to
    A. diagnose dental disease.
    B. look for interproximal caries.
    C. look at the maxillary sinuses.
    D. locate specific dental anomalies.

16. Extraoral radiographs are used by the dentist to identify
    A. overhanging crowns or restorations.
    B. both the mandible and maxilla at the same time.
    C. caries in the anterior teeth.
    D. decay between tooth surfaces.

17. Which of the following could result in a panoramic X-ray with a flat occlusal plane or smile line?
    A. Chin tipped too low
    B. Chin tipped too high
    C. Chin held too far forward
    D. Chin held too far back

18. Digital radiography uses less radiation than film-based radiography because
     A. exposure time is increased.
     B. there is no developing time with digital.
     C. the sensor is larger than the film.
     D. the sensor is more sensitive than film.

See p. 55 for the correct answers and rationales

Processing Radiographs

I. Working with Radiographic Solutions
   A. There are two processing solutions: the developer and the fixer.
      1. The developer is the first chemical in the process. It first softens the gelatin and then interacts with silver halide crystals, leaving black silver specks on the film.
      2. After the developer, the film is briefly rinsed in water and then immersed in a fixer solution. Fixer chemicals halt the development process, wash away any underexposed or unexposed silver halide, and harden the emulsion.
   B. Maintain the integrity of processing solutions.
      1. In manual processing tanks, fixer and developer solutions lose strength over time because of exposure to oxygen. Using a cover prolongs the life of the solutions.
      2. In automatic processing units, processing solutions should be checked every day (in machines without automatic replenishing pumps). Add new solution as necessary. Never use conventional darkroom processing solutions in an automatic processor. The solutions used in automatic processors are ultra concentrated and require additional hardeners and other ingredients. Prepare solutions according to the manufacturer's instructions.

II. Processing Exposed Radiographs
   A. Identify optimum conditions and processes for processing radiographs.
      1. In manual processes, a darkroom should be large enough for one person and be light safe. It should have a safelight, an overhead white light, a viewing safelight, an X-ray view box, sinks, workspace, processing unit and solutions, timer, film hangers, film dryer, and adequate ventilation.
      2. In automatic processes, the unit may require daily, weekly, or monthly cleaning, depending on the manufacturer's specifications. Some units may require that a special cleaning film is fed through every day to remove residue from the rollers. Check processing solutions every day (in machines without automatic replenishing pumps). Add new solution as necessary.
   B. Identify and correct processing errors.
      1. Spots on film can be from chemical contamination, such as the film being in contact with developer or fixer before processing. If so, make sure darkroom surfaces are clean and no chemicals are exposed. They can also come from handling errors, such a low level of developer or fixer. In this case, make sure film is immersed in solution; add solution if necessary.
      2. Fogged film can come from leaks in darkroom conditions, improper safelight, contaminated solutions, exposure to secondary radiation, improper film storage, or a too-hot developer. To prevent this, test for darkroom light tight; check filters and wattage on safe light; do not leave film where they can be exposed to secondary radiation; do not use expired film; do store film in a cool, dry, protected place; and check temperature of developer.
      3. Light images come from weak or cold developing solution or insufficient developing time. Dark images come from excessive developing time, a too-hot developing solution, or a concentrated solution. To correct this, replenish/replace developing solution, correct for proper temperature/working thermometer, and test timer for accuracy.
      4. Clear film comes from being left in the fixer too long or left in a running water bath for 24 or 48 hours. Correct this by timing the fixer solution and never leaving film hanger in running water bath overnight.
      5. Partial images result from a processing error resulting from tanks that are only partially filled.
      6. Stains occur when the operator's hands were contaminated with fluoride. Wash hands thoroughly before handling radiographs.

7. Discolored film occurs when it is not allowed enough time in the fixer bath or the film was not adequately rinsed. Correct this by making sure the film is in the fixer for twice the time as the developer. Rinse for 20 minutes.

8. Loading too many films at once can lead to overlap. Allow at least 10 seconds before each new film to prevent this.

9. Air bubbles occur when air is trapped against the film surface during processing. Correct this by agitating the film hangers when they are first placed into solutions.

C. Identify and correct film handling errors.

1. Scratches look like white lines on film. They occur when the emulsion is scratched, usually by placing one film hanger in the solution alongside a second hanger; they can also be caused by fingernails or any sharp object. Take care never to touch surface of film and discard any broken or damaged film hangers.

2. White lines on film are caused by scratches. Black lines are caused by bending. Bending the film is caused by handling the film so roughly that it is bent.

3. Static electricity looks like black streaks of lightening on film. This occurs when film packets are opened rapidly or before the operator has discharged static charge on his or her skin. To prevent this, discharge any conductive object before handling film.

4. Fingerprints occur when the operator's hands were contaminated with fluoride. Wash hands thoroughly before handling radiographs. Fingerprints can be caused by any touching of the film, so films should only be handled by their edges.

III. Infection Control During Radiographic Processing

A. At the end of an exposure series, the exposed film packets should be swiped across a disinfectant-soaked towel to remove saliva and then transported in a labeled paper cup to a safe area in the office.

B. If disposable plastic film envelopes were used during exposure, the film packets can be safely handled with clean, dry hands or treatment gloves once they've been removed from the envelopes. Care must be taken not to contaminate the daylight loader by inserting films with contaminated gloves.

C. After the film has been placed into the processing tank or automatic film processing unit, aseptic measures should be taken in the darkroom work area.

D. All of the film packets, foil wrappers, cups, and any materials used during transport of the film should be disposed of and the darkroom should be disinfected.

IV. Follow Occupational Safety and Health Administration (OSHA) secondary labeling when storing chemicals.

V. Properly dispose of all chemical agents and other waste materials.

A. Developer and fixer solutions are strong chemicals that should not be poured down a drain after they are exhausted. In many cities, disposal of these chemicals is regulated by law, and dental offices should check with their local waste management company to make sure they are complying with the law when disposing of used solution.

VI. Follow quality assurance procedures when processing radiographs.

Review Questions

19. Insufficient time in the fixer solution will cause films to appear
    A. green.
    B. brown.
    C. clear.
    D. black.

20. What causes reticulation?
    A. The temperature change from developer to rinse water is too great.
    B. The chemicals are exhausted, causing the film to crack.
    C. The emulsion of the film is expired and has cracked.
    D. The developing solution is weak or cold.

21. A step-wedge is used to
    A. determine the film speed.
    B. check the strength of the processing solutions.
    C. identify light leaks in the darkroom.
    D. evaluate safelight adequacy.

22. The ideal temperature for the developing solution is
    A. 58° F.
    B. 68° F.
    C. 74° F.
    D. 80° F.

23. In manual film processing, which of the following steps is done first?
    A. Developing
    B. Fixing
    C. Rinsing
    D. Washing

24. Which automatic processor solution removes the unexposed and undeveloped crystals from the film emulsion?
    A. Developer
    B. Fixer
    C. Replenisher
    D. Water

25. The size of the crystals in the film's emulsion will determine its
    A. film speed.
    B. film type.
    C. image contrast.
    D. image density.

26. A film's exposure to white light during the developing process will cause the image to be
    A. clear.
    B. light.
    C. black.
    D. blurry.

See p. 55 for the correct answers and rationales

Mounting and Labeling Radiographs

I. Mounting Radiographs in the Buccal View
   A. Using anatomical landmarks to orient mounting
      1. Maxillary teeth have larger crowns and longer roots than mandibular teeth. Maxillary molars typically have three molars, but the palatal root makes it difficult to visualize all three roots.
      2. Canine teeth have the longest roots.
      3. Mandibular molars have two roots with visible bone between them. Most roots curve toward the distal.
      4. Large radiolucent areas of the nasal fossa or maxillary sinus indicate a maxillary radiograph.
      5. The mandible has a distinctive upward curve in the molar area. Sometimes called the "smile line," this helps orient radiographs.
      6. Bitewing radiographs should be mounted with the occlusal plane between the mandibular and maxillary teeth (called the curve of Spee) facing upward, toward the distal.
   B. Films are mounted in the appropriate film views to match the anatomic location in the mouth.

C. After processing, dry radiographs should be mounted in holders for better viewing. Mounting should always be done on a clean, light-colored surface to protect the films. This makes it easier to see the radiographs when they are laid out on the worktable. After mounting, films are viewed in a view box or illuminator.

II. Interpreting Radiographs
   A. During interpretation, identify and distinguish any of the following features that might be present on a dental radiograph: normal dental anatomy; abnormal anatomy; restoration, implants, and foreign object; dental caries; periodontal disease, trauma, and lesions.
   B. Black regions on the film are caused by structures that are radiolucent, or structures through which X-rays easily pass, such as soft tissues and open spaces between teeth.
   C. Areas that are more dense, or radiopaque, allow less X-ray energy to get through. These are the white areas on the final radiograph.

III. Legal Issues with Radiographs
   A. Duplications are exact copies of the original radiographs. They can be obtained during exposure by using a two-film packet or after processing by using a film duplicator and duplicating film.
   B. The patient's name, date, and dentist's name must appear on the mount label.
   C. Radiographs are part of a patient's permanent dental record. Dental radiographs, along with the patient's dental history, should be stored indefinitely. When patients switch dental practices and request that their records and radiographs be forwarded to the new dentists, make duplicates of both the dental record and the radiographs.

Review Questions

27. In which exposure would one identify the genial tubercle as a landmark?
    A. Maxillary incisor
    B. Mandibular incisor
    C. Mandibular premolar
    D. Maxillary molar

28. Which of the following landmarks can only be seen on a mandibular exposure?
    A. Incisive foramen
    B. Inverted Y
    C. Mental foramen
    D. Coronoid process

29. Intraoral films should be mounted
    A. next to the patient.
    B. in a clean, wet area.
    C. in the darkroom.
    D. on a light box.

30. The preferred method of film mounting by the ADA is the
    A. anatomical mounting.
    B. dot mounting.
    C. labial mounting.
    D. lingual mounting.

31. What is the purpose of the convex dot on intraoral film?
    A. To identify where to hold the film
    B. To determine film orientation
    C. To identify anatomical landmarks
    D. To mount radiographs in the correct order

See p. 55 for the correct answers and rationales

Radiation Safety for Patients

I. Apply the Principles of Radiation and Health Physics and Hazards

    A. Together, the kVp, mA, and exposure time dictate the characteristics of the X-ray beam. A higher mA, higher kVp, and a longer exposure time equal an increased density. A lower mA, lower kVp, and shorter exposure time equal a decreased density.

        1. X-rays are small wavelength, high-penetrating waves. They are known as ionizing radiation for their ability to ionize molecules, a process that is very damaging to biologic tissues.

    B. X-ray machines have certain safety features.

        1. A metal housing on the outside is lined with lead or made from lead to prevent radiation leakage.

        2. An aluminum filter just outside the X-ray tube filters out the nonpenetrating, longer wavelength beams.

        3. The unit must be outfitted with a collimator that fits over the opening where the X-ray beam emerges from the machine. The collimator must be made from lead and the opening must not be more than 2.75 in in diameter. This limits the radiation emitted to no more than 2.75 in.

        4. The PID is a device on the X-ray tubehead that aims the X-ray beam; PIDs are available in cylindrical and rectangular shapes, with rectangular shapes reducing radiation exposure.

    C. Understand radiation physics.

        1. Primary radiation are X-rays that came directly from the X-ray tube where they are generated. These are high-energy, short-wavelength beams that travel in a straight line from their source. In practice, this is often referred to as the useful beam.

        2. Secondary radiation is created when the X-ray beam interacts with another substance—in this case, the patient's tissues. Secondary radiation has less energy and longer wavelengths than primary radiation. It is not considered useful because it creates foggy or cloudy dental radiographs.

    D. If malfunction of the X-ray machine is suspected, alert the dentist, and do not take any more radiographs until the machine is deemed safe.

II. Patient Radiographic Safety Practices

    A. Unnecessary x-radiation exposure comes from secondary radiation, scatter radiation, and leakage radiation.

    B. Radiation causes biologic damage through ionization. X-rays are frequently called ionizing radiation because of their ability to interact with, and change, atoms. Thus, X-rays are capable of changing molecular structures in the body, affecting organ tissues.

        1. Damage occurs when individuals are either exposed to high levels of radiation suddenly (e.g., acute exposure) or exposed to low levels of radiation over a very long time (e.g., chronic exposure). Acute exposure can cause immediate cell death. At lower levels, the effect on cells, and therefore health, depends on the cell type. Radiation exposure can cause damage to the DNA located within somatic cells. Cell division may be prevented or compromised, resulting in damage to the organism. In contrast, genetic cells experience damage to the chromosomes carried within the cells and can be passed to future generations.

        2. The period between radiation exposure and its biological effect is the latent period, which can be several years.

    C. ALARA stands for "as low as reasonably achievable." This means exposing patients and operators to the lowest possible dose of radiation that will get the job done. Dental radiographs should never be prescribed on a routine basis and should be based on clinical need. Today, most state regulatory agencies require documentation of need rather than radiographs being taken routinely.

    D. Before any radiographs are ordered, a complete oral examination should be conducted and a patient history should be taken, including any medical conditions as well as previous exposure to X-rays. This information should weigh into the decision to prescribe X-ray imaging. Indications for dental radiographs include history of previous dental disease, positive clinical signs/symptoms, and increased risk of dental caries.

Review Questions

32. What types of cells are most easily destroyed or altered?
    A. Bone cells
    B. Brain cells
    C. Blood-forming cells
    D. Nerve cells

33. A collimator is used to
    A. reduce the size of the primary beam.
    B. remove attenuated radiation.
    C. minimize patient exposure time.
    D. filter scatter radiation.

34. What do the letters in ALARA mean?
    A. As low as reasonably achievable
    B. As low as reasonably available
    C. As long as roentgens approved
    D. As long as reasonably available

35. What kind of radiation exposure causes damage slowly over time before the effects are noticed?
    A. Acute
    B. Chronic
    C. Cumulative
    D. Natural

36. The use of a thyroid collar is contraindicated when exposing
    A. panoramic radiographs.
    B. occlusal radiographs.
    C. intraoral films on children.
    D. intraoral films on edentulous patients.

37. If the dental assistant suspects that the X-ray machine is malfunctioning, which of the following actions should be taken?
    A. Adjust the collimator and continue with the series.
    B. Check the machine at the end of the day.
    C. Immediately stop exposures and notify the dentist.
    D. Submit a written report to the office manager.

38. The ADA guidelines recommend that radiographs should be taken how often?
    A. Every 6 months
    B. Every 12 to 18 months
    C. Once every 2 years
    D. As necessary

39. What is another name for secondary radiation?
    A. Controlled
    B. Short
    C. Scatter
    D. Thermoluminescent

40. All of the following cause unnecessary radiation exposure EXCEPT
    A. re-takes.
    B. optimum film processing.
    C. slow-speed film.
    D. scatter radiation.

41. Erythema, nausea, diarrhea, hemorrhage, and loss of hair are signs and symptoms seen with
    A. long-term effects of radiation.
    B. short-term effects of radiation.
    C. cataracts.
    D. primary radiation.

42. Which of the following components of the tubehead helps reduce X-ray exposure?
    A. X-ray tube
    B. Metal housing
    C. Oil bath
    D. Step-up transformer

43. Which of the following would result in the LEAST radiation exposure to the patient?
    A. Slow film speed and high kVp
    B. Slow film speed and low kVp
    C. Fast film speed and low kVp
    D. Fast film speed and high kVp

See p. 55 for the correct answers and rationales

Radiation Safety for Dental Staff

I. Operator Radiographic Safety Practices
   A. Repeated use of X-rays raises the risk of cumulative, long-term exposure to scatter or secondary radiation, and poorly sealed X-ray units can expose assistants to leakage radiation.
   B. Identify safety measures to reduce operator risk.
      1. Limit exposure whenever possible.
      2. Never try to stabilize patients or the X-ray device manually.
      3. Never hold an X-ray tube manually because leaked radiation can dramatically increase exposure.
      4. Take care to shield yourself from X-rays. Most dentists' offices are built with some form of structural shielding where you can take refuge during exposure. If shielding is not an option—for example, in an older practice with open bays—remain as far away as possible from the X-ray unit. Ideally, stand at least 6 feet away, behind the bulkiest part of the patient's head, and between 90 degrees and 135 degrees out of the primary beam.
   C. The risk for X-ray operators is somewhat different than the risk for patients because X-ray operators are not exposed to the primary radiation. However, repeated use of X-rays raises the risk of cumulative, long-term exposure to scatter or secondary radiation, and poorly sealed X-ray units can expose you to leakage radiation. Scatter radiation is a form of secondary radiation in which the direction of travel has been changed. In addition, radiation exposure can be reduced with periodic inspection of X-ray equipment and periodic wearing of a dosimeter.
II. Monitoring Personal Radiation Exposure
   A. The ALARA concept was designed to help people understand how to approach radiation. ALARA stands for "as low as reasonably achievable." In practice, this means exposing patients and operators to the lowest possible dose of radiation that will get the job done. Dental radiographs should never be prescribed on a routine basis. Their use should be based on clinical need. Today, most state regulatory agencies require documentation of need rather than radiographs being taken routinely.

Radiation Health and Safety

B. Personal monitoring devices alert the operator that he or she has been exposed to radiation. A number of devices are available and the various devices measure different factors. Some will only tell if radiation exposure had occurred, some will tell what kind of radiation exposure has occurred, and some will measure both the kind and the dose.

Review Questions

44. Coulomb per kilogram (C/kg) is equivalent to which unit of exposure that is used in the United States?
    A. roentgen (R)
    B. RAD
    C. REM
    D. Sievert (Sv)

45. What is used to determine the amount of radiation exposure an operator has received?
    A. A dosimeter badge
    B. A blood test
    C. The number of radiographs exposed
    D. The MPD formula

46. The time frame between exposure to radiation and development of biologic effects is called the
    A. radiosensitive period.
    B. sievert period.
    C. latent period.
    D. rad period.

47. What is the maximum dosage of radiation for a dental assistant per year?
    A. 0.1 REM
    B. 0.5 REM
    C. 5 REMs
    D. 10 REMs

48. Which of the following choices is the BEST way to take a periapical radiograph on an uncooperative 5-year-old child?
    A. The clinician holds the film during exposure.
    B. The parent holds the film during exposure.
    C. The radiograph is taken when the child is older.
    D. The clinician takes a panoramic radiograph instead.

49. When exposing a radiograph, the operator should stand
    A. at least 6 feet away from the X-ray beam.
    B. only at right angles to the tubehead.
    C. in front of the patient to monitor film position.
    D. next to the patient while wearing a lead apron.

See p. 55 for the correct answers and rationales

ANSWERS AND RATIONALES:
Radiation Health and Safety

Expose and Evaluate

1. What characteristic will a radiograph exhibit if the film was placed backward in the mouth?

   C. Herringbone effect. A film placed backward will have a herringbone effect and appear lighter.

2. Elongation on a dental radiograph is caused by

   D. too little vertical angle. Elongation results from insufficient vertical angulation in the bisecting technique.

3. When taking a radiograph of a 6-year-old patient, which of the following adjustments is made for the child's size?

   C. Shorter exposure time. Exposure time is reduced to compensate for the smaller bone mass and tissue density of a child.

4. Cone cutting results when the central ray

   A. is not aimed at the center of the film. In order for the entire film to be exposed, the PID is placed so that it completely covers the film on all sides. The central ray, an imaginary line through the center or the PID, should strike in the middle of the film.

5. If the focal-film distance, or FFD, is increased and the mA remains the same, the image will have

   A. decreased magnification. Film magnification causes image distortion, and the goal is to decrease it as much as possible. Placing the film as close as possible to the tooth (or target) reduces magnification and increases image sharpness.

6. Penumbra is the

   D. diffuse outline of the image. Penumbra is a partial shadow around an object.

7. Which of the following positioning errors results in an overlapped image?

   C. Incorrect horizontal angulation. Overlapped images result when the central beam fails to pass directly through the interproximal spaces of the teeth in the horizontal plane.

8. When using an aiming ring to align the PID, the rim on the open end of the tube should be

   A. parallel to the ring. Using the paralleling technique, the alignment ring, the open end of the PID, and the sensor should all be parallel to each other.

9. Overlapping the contact areas on a bitewing radiograph is an indication that the

    A. horizontal angulation is off. Proper horizontal angulation of an exposure will project the central ray through the contacts of the teeth in the film. If horizontal angulation is off, then the contacts will appear overlapped and the film will not be diagnostic.

10. Filters are used in the X-ray tubehead to reduce

    D. the patient radiation dose. Aluminum filters are used to remove low energy, long wavelength X-rays from the beam. These X-rays are harmful to the patient and not useful in exposing the image.

11. How should film be repositioned when the third molar is not showing up on a radiograph of the mandibular molar area?

    D. Move the film farther back in the mouth. The film needs to be positioned farther back in the mouth (moved distally), so that the image of the third molar will be included on the film.

12. The distal surface of the canine should be observed in which of the following radiograph exposures?

    B. Premolar bitewing. When the film is properly placed, the distal of the canine should appear on the premolar periapical or the premolar bitewing.

13. Which of the following anatomical landmarks is not visible in the mandibular molar exposure?

    B. Mental foramen. The mental foramen is visible near the apices of the mandibular first and second premolar and will not be visible in the molar exposure.

14. The horizontal line from the top of the ear through the corner of the eye that is used for positioning a patient for a panoramic film is the

    C. Frankfort plane. The Frankfort plane is determined by visualizing a line from the top of the patient's ear horizontally through the corner of the eye. In order to line a patient up properly for a quality panoramic exposure, the Frankfort plane should be parallel to the floor.

15. Occlusal radiographs are used to

    D. locate specific dental anomalies. The occlusal exposure is used to visualize large areas of the arches to identify the location of different anomalies, such as supernumerary teeth, fractures, pulp stones, and areas of clefting.

16. Extraoral radiographs are used by the dentist to identify

    C. caries in the anterior teeth. The purpose of the extraoral exposure, such as the panoramic, is to allow the dentist to view the entire dentition and surround structures.

17. Which of the following could result in a panoramic X-ray with a flat occlusal plane or smile line?

    B. Chin tipped too high. The chin should be positioned so that the ala-tragus line is parallel with the floor.

18. Digital radiography uses less radiation than film-based radiography because

> **D. the sensor is more sensitive than film.** The digital sensor is much more sensitive to radiation than film. It takes less than one quarter of the amount of radiation to take a digital exposure than to take a film-based exposure.

Processing Radiographs

19. Insufficient time in the fixer solution will cause films to appear

> **B. brown.** Films that are removed from the fixer solution before the recommended time will appear foggy and have a brown tint to them.

20. What causes reticulation?

> **A. The temperature change from developer to rinse water is too great.** Reticulation occurs when the film is exposed to an extreme change in temperature from the developer to the water bath. All solutions should be the same temperature.

21. A step-wedge is used to

> **B. check the strength of the processing solutions.** The step-wedge is used to check the strength/quality of the processing solutions, as well as monitoring the consistency of radiation output of the X-ray machine.

22. The ideal temperature for the developing solution is

> **B. 68° F.** At 68° F, films should be developed for 5 minutes. Any temperature above 68° F will require a shorter developing time and any temperature below 68° F will require a longer developing time.

23. In manual film processing, which of the following steps is done first?

> **A. Developing.** The correct sequence for manual film processing is developing, rinsing, fixing, and washing.

24. Which automatic processor solution removes the unexposed and undeveloped crystals from the film emulsion?

> **B. Fixer.** Sodium thiosulfate or ammonium thiosulfate in the fixer solution removes all unexposed, undeveloped silver halide crystals from emulsion.

25. The size of the crystals in the film's emulsion will determine its

> **A. film speed.** The silver halide crystals in the emulsion will determine the speed of the film. The larger the silver halide crystals, the faster the film speeds will be.

26. A film's exposure to white light during the developing process will cause the image to be

> **C. black.** If there is a white light leak in the darkroom or daylight loader, the finished film will appear foggy or black, depending on the severity of the light leak.

Radiation Health and Safety

Mounting and Labeling Radiographs

27. In which exposure would one identify the genial tubercle as a landmark?

   B. Mandibular incisor. The genial tubercle is a radiopaque, donut-shaped area that surrounds the lingual foramen.

28. Which of the following landmarks can only be seen on a mandibular exposure?

   C. Mental foramen. The mental foramen appears near the apex of the mandibular first premolar.

29. Intraoral films should be mounted

   D. on a light box. Radiographs are best viewed on a light box in a dim room.

30. The preferred method of film mounting by the ADA is the

   C. labial mounting. The ADA recommends that operators use the labial mounting method of organizing radiographs. The identification dot is raised and should face the outer surface of the mount.

31. What is the purpose of the convex dot on intraoral film?

   B. To determine film orientation. A tiny embossed dot is used to help orient the film, so that all the films are placed into a mount facing the same way.

Radiation Safety for Patients

32. What types of cells are most easily destroyed or altered?

   C. Blood-forming cells. Blood-forming cells are the most sensitive and easiest to be destroyed.

33. A collimator is used to

   A. reduce the size of the primary beam. The collimator is used to restrict the size and shape of the X-ray beam. It may be round or rectangular and will assist in reducing patients' exposure to radiation.

34. What do the letters in ALARA mean?

   A. As low as reasonably achievable. The ALARA concept stands for *as low as reasonably achievable*. This means that the patient should be exposed to the absolute least amount of radiation needed to accomplish the outcome.

35. What kind of radiation exposure causes damage slowly over time before the effects are noticed?

   C. Cumulative. In cumulative exposure, cell damage slowly builds up, sometimes for years, before effects become known.

36. The use of a thyroid collar is contraindicated when exposing

   A. panoramic radiographs. When using rotational panoramic equipment, the use of a thyroid collar may obscure diagnostic information or interfere with the rotation of the panoramic X-ray unit.

37. If the dental assistant suspects that the X-ray machine is malfunctioning, which of the following actions should be taken?

   C. Immediately stop exposures and notify the dentist. A malfunctioning X-ray unit could cause unnecessary radiation exposure to the patient and the operator, so if there is a suspected problem, all exposures should stop, and the dentist should be notified.

38. The ADA guidelines recommend that radiographs should be taken how often?

   D. As necessary. The ADA recommends that radiographs be taken based on the patient's individual health needs. Because each patient is different from the next, the scheduling of X-ray exams must be individualized for each patient.

39. What is another name for secondary radiation?

   C. Scatter. Scatter radiation is the secondary radiation produced when the primary radiation beam strikes the patient and bounces off in another direction.

40. All of the following cause unnecessary radiation exposure EXCEPT

   B. optimum film processing. Optimum film processing reduces re-takes of radiographs, minimizing unnecessary radiation. Re-takes, slow film speed, and scatter radiation cause unnecessary radiation exposure to the patient

41. Erythema, nausea, diarrhea, hemorrhage, and loss of hair are signs and symptoms seen with

   B. short-term effects of radiation. Short-term effects of radiation include erythema, nausea, diarrhea, hemorrhage, and loss of hair. Redness or erythema is the first clinical sign of acute radiation toxicity.

42. Which of the following components of the tubehead helps reduce X-ray exposure?

   B. Metal housing. A metal housing on the outside of the tubehead is lined with lead or made from lead to prevent radiation leakage.

43. Which of the following would result in the LEAST radiation exposure to the patient?

   D. Fast film speed and high kVp. Fast film speed reduces the time the patient is exposed to radiation and a high kVp increases the number of short, penetrating X-rays that are able to reach the target tissues.

Radiation Safety for Dental Staff

44. Coulomb per kilogram (C/kg) is equivalent to which unit of exposure that is used in the United States?

    A. roentgen (R). Coulomb per kilogram converts to the roentgen in the United States. A roentgen is the amount of radiation it takes to produce 1 esu of electricity in 1 cc of air

45. What is used to determine the amount of radiation exposure an operator has received?

    A. A dosimeter badge. A dosimeter badge is worn for a predetermined period of time and then evaluated for exposure.

46. The time frame between exposure to radiation and development of biologic effects is called the

    C. latent period. Most exposures to radiation are received over a period of time before any measurable damage is noted. This is referred to as a latent period.

47. What is the maximum dosage of radiation for a dental assistant per year?

    C. 5 REMs. No more than 5 REMs is allowable for the dental assistant in a year.

48. Which of the following choices is the BEST way to take a periapical radiograph on an uncooperative 5-year-old child?

    B. The parent holds the film during exposure. The best way to gain cooperation from a young child is to enlist the help of a parent. Both parent and child should utilize lead aprons. Clinicians should never hold films and expose themselves to unnecessary radiation.

49. When exposing a radiograph, the operator should stand

    A. at least 6 feet away from the X-ray beam. For safety reasons, the operator should stand out of the way of the primary bean. Ideally, there would be a lead lined wall or shield for the operator to stand behind. If there is not, then the operator must stand at least 6 feet away from the tubehead.

INFECTION CONTROL (ICE)

Patient and Dental Healthcare Worker Education

I. Infectious Diseases and Their Relationship to Patient Safety and Occupational Risk
  A. An infection occurs when diseases-causing organisms, known as pathogens, cause illness. Infections can be local infections, confined to a single area or region of the body, or they can be systemic infections, present throughout the body. Skin infections are common local infections. Systemic infections include most viruses and some dangerous bacterial infections. A number of organisms can cause infection: bacteria, viruses, protozoa, fungi, and prions.
  B. Infection control is a routine part of all modern dental practices. According to the principle of standard precautions, all patients are treated as if they are potentially infectious. This means that all blood is treated as if it is harboring HIV, hepatitis, or other infectious organisms. Universal precautions are valuable for two reasons. The first is that it is often impossible to tell by sight alone if a patient is potentially infected—and not all patients always give accurate information in their medical histories. The second is it prevents legal complications that might occur when dental offices discriminate between one class of patients as potentially infectious and another as "safer."

II. Explain and Clarify Procedures, Services, and Consequences
  A. Provide information to the patient about the importance of following infection control protocol during delivery of dental care to protect the patient's health and the health of the dental team.

III. Immunizing Against Infectious Diseases
  A. Immunizations are a standard part of infection control. In the dental office, only hepatitis B vaccination is covered by Occupational Safety and Health Administration (OSHA) regulation. According to OSHA, all employees must be offered the hepatitis B vaccination within 10 days of starting employment. Medical professionals are also recommended to receive vaccination against influenza.

Infection Control

Review Questions

1. Which airborne infectious disease is a leading cause of death worldwide and is an occupational risk for healthcare workers?
    A. HIV
    B. Legionnaires' disease
    C. Tetanus
    D. Tuberculosis

2. A pandemic disease is one that
    A. is temporary.
    B. is characterized by immediate symptoms.
    C. occurs over a large geographic area.
    D. occurs in a specific population only.

3. Which type of hepatitis is spread through the fecal-oral route?
    A. Hepatitis A
    B. Hepatitis B
    C. Hepatitis C
    D. Hepatitis D

4. Dental employers are required to maintain accurate medical records on their employees who are at risk for contamination from bloodborne pathogens. These records are to be kept
    A. until the employee leaves the position.
    B. as long as the employer is in practice.
    C. as long as the employee remains in the profession.
    D. the length of employment plus 30 years.

5. Which of the following items is classified as semicritical?
    A. Bur
    B. Scaler
    C. Lead apron
    D. Rubber dam forceps

See p. 71 for the correct answers and rationales

Standard Precautions to Prevent Disease Transmission

I. Prevent Cross-Contamination and Disease Transmission
   A. Wash hands with a non-antimicrobial or antimicrobial soap and water when hands are visibly dirty or contaminated with blood or other potentially infectious material. Also, wash hands after barehanded touching of inanimate objects likely to be contaminated by blood, saliva, or respiratory secretions and before and after gloving for each patient. If hands are not visibly soiled, use an alcohol-based hand rub.
   B. Use one-time-use (unit dose), disposable supplies, which are an excellent way to prevent cross-contamination. These supplies are frequently made from paper, plastic, or light metal.
   C. Cover anything that can become potentially contaminated with a protective barrier: handles, knobs, counter surfaces, faucets, handpieces, air-water syringes, high-volume evacuators, saliva ejectors, pens and pencils, and tubing. Protective barriers are often made of disposable plastic, and special products have been introduced that conform to hard-to-cover areas, such as the tubing that connects the air-water syringe. Change protective barriers between every patient and disposed of them in a safe manner.

II. Maintenance of Asepsis
   A. The chain of infection describes the steps that a microbe takes as it travels from one host to another.
      1. An infectious agent is a microbe, such as bacteria, viruses, protozoa, or fungi.
      2. A reservoir is a hospitable environment for an infectious agent to thrive and multiply, such as people.
      3. A portal of exit is the vehicle by which the infectious agent leaves the reservoir and travels to a new host, such as a nostril.
      4. A mode of transmission is the method by which the infectious agent moves from the portal of exit to the new host, such as direct or indirect transmission, airborne transmission, or parenteral transmission.
      5. A portal of entry is the means of entry into the body, such as oral and nasal cavities.
      6. A susceptible host is any organism that can provide a suitable environment for an infectious agent to thrive, such as a person.
   B. Properly dispose of biohazardous and other waste.
      1. Sterilize extracted teeth before they are disposed of or given to patients. However, if teeth contain amalgams, they should not be sterilized due to toxic vapors and must be disposed of as biohazardous waste.
      2. Sharps are regulated waste; store them in clearly marked sharps containers and dispose them with an agency that specializes in sharp disposal.
      3. Radiographic supplies are regulated waste; dispose of them according to federal and local guidelines.
      4. Dental amalgam contains mercury, which is highly toxic. Store amalgam waste in a clearly marked container in the dental office and use a mercury disposal company to dispose of it.
      5. The handling of chemicals in the dental office is governed by OSHA's Hazard Communication Standard.
   C. Keep instruments wrapped in sterilization packages in their packages until they are opened to be used. Store intact packages of sterilized instruments in a clean, dry, and cool place.

III. Procedures for Sterilizing Instruments and Equipment

    A. Preparations for sterilization.

        1. Process contaminated instruments either immediately or place them into a holding solution until attention can be paid to them. The first step in the sterilization procedure is to preclean the instruments. This typically includes ultrasonic cleaning or cleaning in an approved automatic washer.

        2. After use with a patient, wipe handpieces clean of visible debris and attach them to the unit with a bur in place. Run it briefly to flush out the lines of any water, air, and debris. Take it back to the sterilization area, where it can be cleaned and sterilized according to the manufacturer's instructions.

    B. Use the appropriate method for sterilization/disinfection.

        1. High-level disinfection is used for objects that cannot withstand heat sterilization, such as rubber dam guides and X-ray film holding devices.

        2. Low-temperature sterilization can also be accomplished in an ethylene oxide sterilization unit.

        3. Dry heat sterilization accomplishes sterilization by exposing instruments to temperatures of at least 320° to 375° F for 1 hour. It can be used with loose or packaged instruments but no plastics, fabrics, or rubber.

        4. Chemical vapor sterilizers create a sterilizing fog from chemicals like alcohol or formaldehyde. The lack of water vapor inside the unit means that metals and other materials will not corrode as rapidly.

        5. Steam sterilization uses pressurized steam to rapidly sterilize both wrapped and unwrapped instruments.

        6. To sterilize a handpiece, closely follow the manufacturer's instructions. Handpieces can be sterilized in steam units in the appropriate packaging.

    C. Use the appropriate system for monitoring and sterilization of instruments and equipment.

        1. Biologic monitoring, or live spore testing, uses samples of specially prepared samples of spores of nonpathogenic microorganisms to test the effectiveness of sterilization. A control is always used and spore growth indicates that sterilization has not occurred. Any positive spore test requires that instruments be resterilized and tested again. If still positive, the sterilizer should not be used until it has been checked. A negative test indicates that the sterilization unit is not working as it should.

        2. Chemical monitoring uses special chemical labels or inks that react with the sterilization environment. It is useful on a day-to-day basis to confirm that the conditions required for sterilization were present. There are two kinds of chemical monitoring: process indicators, used on the outside of sterilization packages; and dosage indicators, used in sterilization units that rely on chemical vapors at certain concentrations, dry heat, or steam.

IV. Cleaning, Disinfecting, and Protecting the Dental Environment

    A. Surfaces must always be precleaned before disinfection to ensure maximum effectiveness of the disinfectant.

    B. Use the proper method to disinfect the treatment room, laboratory, instrument processing, and equipment.

        1. To disinfect the treatment room, prepare the cleaning solution. Make sure instrument trays and immersion baths with instruments have been taken to the sterilization area. Remove all physical barriers. Spray disinfectant directly onto a cotton gauze or use premoistened disinfectant wipes.

        2. Avoid cross-contamination and exercise infection control measures in the laboratory as you would in the treatment area. Disinfect the laboratory area and any contaminated items or equipment after each use.

        3. After the film has been placed into the processing tank or automatic film processing unit, aseptic measures should be taken in the darkroom. All of the film packets, foil wrappers, cups, and any materials used during transport of the film should be disposed of, and the darkroom should be disinfected. Surface disinfection should be accomplished on all work areas, including anywhere that was touched with gloved hands.

        4. Equipment is disinfected the same way as the treatment room. Intraoral bite blocks should be sterilized or covered with barriers (digital sensors).

    C. It is important to use disinfectant products exactly according to label instructions. For example, if a product must sit on a surface for 10 to 15 seconds to be effective, users should make sure to include this time in their disinfecting regimen.

    D. Wherever possible, clinical contact surfaces should be protected by physical barriers, such as disposable plastic wrap that is changed between patients. Touch surfaces and transfer surfaces should be disinfected between patients. Splash, spatter, and droplet surfaces should be cleaned and disinfected at least every day.

Review Questions

Prevent Cross-Contamination and Transmission

6. Which of the following OSHA standards is written to protect dental healthcare workers from occupational exposure to infectious diseases?
    A. Hazardous Communication Standard
    B. Universal Precaution Standard
    C. Bloodborne Pathogen Standard
    D. Exposure Control Standard

7. To maintain high filterability, a face mask that is moist from exhaled air should be replaced
    A. every 20 minutes.
    B. every 30 minutes.
    C. every hour.
    D. when saturated.

8. Which of the following personal protective barriers should ALWAYS be put on last?
    A. Gloves
    B. Mask
    C. Protective eyewear
    D. Protective clothing

9. Which of the following is NOT recommended for use as a surface barrier?
    A. Plastic-backed patient napkins
    B. Paper tray liners
    C. Plastic bags
    D. Clear plastic wrap

10. Gloves contaminated during dental procedures should be discarded in the
    A. regular waste receptacle.
    B. regulated medical waste receptacle.
    C. biohazard receptacle.
    D. sharps container.

11. An alcohol-based hand rub should be used only
    A. when sterile gloves are to be donned immediately afterward.
    B. following handwashing with another antimicrobial hand soap.
    C. if there is no visible soil on the hands.
    D. when the hands are visibly soiled.

12. Personal protective equipment includes all of the following EXCEPT
    A. safety glasses with eye shields or face shields.
    B. masks or respirators.
    C. gowns laundered at home.
    D. gloves.

13. Which of the following is NOT true regarding the use of overgloves?
    A. They are acceptable alone as a hand barrier for intraoral procedures.
    B. They are discarded after a single use.
    C. They can be worn over contaminated treatment gloves.
    D. They can be used to touch a noncontaminated object.

14. Which of the following is the BEST way to clean the high-speed handpiece after patient treatment?
    A. Flush 20 to 30 seconds between patients
    B. Sterilize in packaging materials
    C. Place in cold sterile solution overnight
    D. Wipe down with glutaraldehyde solution between patients

15. When performing a thorough hand washing before gloving, you should rinse your hands with water at what temperature?
    A. Cool
    B. Tepid
    C. Warm
    D. Hot

Maintain Aseptic Conditions

16. The front desk and walls of the dental office are classified as housekeeping surfaces and should be cleaned with a
    A. low-level disinfectant.
    B. mid-level disinfectant.
    C. high-level disinfectant.
    D. liquid sterilant.

17. To ensure sterilization, steam sterilizers should be loaded so that
    A. instrument packages completely fill the autoclave.
    B. instrument packages are processed one at a time.
    C. instrument packages are packed loosely into the autoclave.
    D. instrument packages are double wrapped.

18. Dental instruments that are used in the mouth but do not penetrate tissue or bone are
    A. critical instrument.
    B. semicritical instruments.
    C. noncritical instruments.
    D. nonsterile instruments.

19. Improperly cleaning a dental unit after a procedure could lead to what route of cross-contamination?
    A. Patient to staff
    B. Staff to patient
    C. Patient to patient
    D. Office to community

20. Which of the following types of waste must be identified with a biohazard label?
    A. General waste
    B. Hazardous waste
    C. Regulated waste
    D. Chemical waste

Perform Sterilization Procedures

21. When evaluating the effectiveness of the sterilizer, what is used as the test medium?
    A. Fungal protoplasts
    B. Viral capsids
    C. Bacterial endospore
    D. Protozal membranes

22. After being used for patient treatment and before being sterilized, dental instruments should be
    A. soaked in soapy water for 30 minutes.
    B. scrubbed with a brush under running water.
    C. placed straight into a bag and sealed.
    D. placed in the ultrasonic unit or instrument washer.

23. One of the most common liquid sterilants is
    A. glutaraldehyde.
    B. phenol.
    C. sodium hypochlorite.
    D. quaternary ammonium.

24. Which method of sterilization is used for instruments that are subject to corrosion?
    A. Dry heat sterilization
    B. Steam under pressure
    C. Chemical vapor under pressure
    D. High-level chemical disinfection

25. Sterilization is defined as
    A. the reduction of pathogenic microorganisms to a safe level.
    B. the destruction of all life forms.
    C. a cleaning process to enhance disinfection.
    D. the destruction of all bacterial spores.

26. What is the main disadvantage of a chemical vapor sterilizer?
    A. It requires 6 to 10 hours operating time.
    B. It cannot sterilize plastics and fabrics.
    C. It must be placed in a well-ventilated area.
    D. It causes wear and tear on the instruments.

27. Which of the following is the BEST method of preparing instrument packs for the steam autoclave sterilizer?
    A. Environmental Protection Agency (EPA)-approved packaging materials
    B. Centers for Disease Control and Prevention (CDC)-approved packaging materials
    C. Food and Drug Administration (FDA)-approved packaging materials
    D. Health Insurance Portability and Accountability Act (HIPAA)-approved packaging materials

28. When the color indicator on the sterilization package changes color after processing, this indicates that the sterilizer
    A. operated for the correct time frame.
    B. finished sterilizing the instruments.
    C. reached the correct temperature.
    D. reached the correct pressure.

Environmental Asepsis

29. A good way to reduce cross-contamination of dental materials is to use
    A. a disinfectant ahead of time.
    B. disposable materials.
    C. the spray-wipe-spray technique.
    D. materials that have been sterilized before use.

30. Any time a chemical is dispensed into a nonoriginal container, that container should be
    A. marked with a secondary label.
    B. breakproof and sealable.
    C. looked up in the material safety data sheet (MSDS) book.
    D. stored at an alternate site.

31. How long should dental impressions be sterilized before the impression is poured?
    A. 10 minutes
    B. 15 minutes
    C. 20 minutes
    D. 25 minutes

32. The best way to minimize cross-contamination of X-ray equipment is to
    A. use the spray-wipe-spray technique.
    B. double glove before touching.
    C. cover the control panel with plastic.
    D. take off gloves prior to exposing the film.

33. Which of the following chemicals is a high-level disinfectant?
    A. Alcohol
    B. Chlorine dioxide
    C. Iodophor
    D. Sodium hypochlorite

34. The active ingredient in chlorine compounds used in dentistry for intermediate-level surface disinfection is
    A. dimethyl benzyl ammonium chloride.
    B. ethyl alcohol.
    C. iodine.
    D. sodium hypochlorite.

35. Which of the following is the best description of an intermediate-level disinfectant?
    A. Kills most tuberculosis spores and most viruses
    B. Kills all tuberculosis spores and all viruses
    C. Kills some tuberculosis spores and some viruses
    D. Kills all tuberculosis spores and most viruses

36. Which of the following solutions is best for cleaning the dental suction lines?
    A. Bleach, detergent, and water solution
    B. Nondetergent, enzymatic cleaning solution
    C. Detergent, nonenzymatic cleaning solution
    D. Iodophors, detergent, and water cleaning solution

See p. 71 for the correct answers and rationales

Occupational Safety in the Dental Office

I. Occupational Safety for Dental Office Personnel
   A. OSHA's Bloodborne Pathogen Standard (BBP) is a comprehensive protocol designed to protect employees from bloodborne illness. It regulates the use of sharps and exposure incidents to possibly contaminated blood.
      1. All potentially infectious materials, such as blood and saliva, should be considered infectious.
      2. Employees should wash hands immediately following glove removal.
      3. Needles should never be recapped, bent, or broken.
      4. Efforts should be made to minimize splashing of blood and potentially infectious materials.
      5. Employees should wear protective equipment including eye protection and gloves. All employees should be trained when they are hired. Training should be repeated yearly.
      6. Occupational exposure plan must be developed for each workplace and updated yearly.
   B. Follow the regulations in the Hazard Communication Standard (HCS).
      1. Employers must alert employees about hazardous chemicals used in the workplace and develop a hazard communication program.

Infection Control

    2. New employees must be trained in the use and handling of hazardous chemicals within 30 days of beginning employment and once a year after that.

    3. A certificate of training must be kept within the employee's personnel file.

    4. Elements of the HCS include a: chemical inventory form; a material safety data sheet (MSDS); and labeling of all chemicals with quantity, physical state, and hazard class, among other elements.

  C. Follow the OSHA General Work Place Standard.

    1. Give first aid appropriately.

    2. Report and document all infection exposure and first aid incidents

  D. Follow standard guidelines to prevent injuries from needlesticks and other sharps.

II. Safety Measures for Chemical and Physical Hazards

  A. Dental amalgam contains mercury, which is highly toxic. Amalgam waste must be stored in a clearly marked container in the dental office and disposed of by a mercury disposal company.

  B. The maximum allowable amount of nitrous oxide (N_2O) released into the treatment area is 50 parts per million. Occupational risk can be avoided by using a scavenger system, which reduces the N_2O that escapes and is inhaled. Also make sure the patient's nosepiece or mask fits firmly and discourage patients from talking during gas administration, inspect equipment and hoses for leaks, and vent gas outside the building.

  C. When working with chemicals, follow OSHA's HCS.

    1. In the event of a chemical spill, consult the MSDS or product label immediately to learn the best way to clean it up.

    2. Wear chemical-resistant utility gloves when handling toxic material and always wear protective eye wear.

    3. If a chemical accidentally gets into the eye, OSHA requires that all workplaces that use chemicals have eye wash stations.

    4. Other items of protective clothing include gowns, jackets, or rubber and neoprene aprons.

    5. The aprons are recommended when mixing corrosive chemicals or working in the darkroom.

    6. Never handle broken glass because of the risk of tear or puncture wound. Instead, glass should be swept into a dustpan or onto a sheet of cardboard and then disposed of in the sharps container.

    7. When working with laundry, always wear gloves and place laundry into a container that is clearly labeled with the biohazard label.

  D. A well-ventilated office has less fumes, particles, and dust floating in the air, so there is less opportunity to inhale dangerous chemicals. Even small spaces, such as darkrooms, should be adequately ventilated if chemicals are in use. For example, after chemical vapor sterilization, toxic chemicals are released into the environment, potentially causing irritation. Good ventilation is essential and any dental personnel exposed to these devices should wear monitoring badges that measure exposure to airborne chemicals.

  E. The chemical inventory is a complete list of all the hazardous chemicals used in the office. This list should include cleaners and disinfectants, sterilants, composites and bonding material, amalgam, impression agents, and anything that might pose a threat.

  F. Eye wear should also be worn when working with curing lights or lasers because these devices can cause damage to the eyes.

  G. Some chemicals can react with latex, so chemical-resistant utility gloves should be worn when handling toxic material.

  H. Use caution when handling handpieces, lights, or endodontic instruments producing large amounts of heat.

III. A comprehensive quality control system for assuring optimum infection control procedures should be documented and maintained.

Review Questions

37. What should you use to remove needles from reusable syringes?
    A. Hemostat
    B. Gloved hands
    C. Recapping device
    D. Retractor

38. By law, who provides MSDSs for the office?
    A. Dentist
    B. Manufacturer
    C. OSHA
    D. Vendor

39. It is important for the dental assistant to have a foundation in microbiology in order to
    A. cure disease in the dental setting.
    B. prevent disease transmission in the dental setting.
    C. diagnose disease transmission in the dental setting.
    D. evaluate disease transmission in the dental setting.

40. The purpose of OSHA is to protect whom?
    A. Consumers
    B. Employees
    C. Employers
    D. The public

41. Utilizing universal/standard precautions is enforced by the
    A. CDC.
    B. EPA.
    C. ADA.
    D. OSHA.

42. Which agent is NOT recommended by the CDC for surface disinfection?
    A. Sodium hypochlorite
    B. Ethyl alcohol
    C. Phenols
    D. Glutaraldehyde

43. An office exposure control program must be updated
    A. monthly.
    B. biannually.
    C. annually.
    D. as changes occur.

44. If an employee is stuck with a needle or contaminated instrument, the employee should remove his/her gloves then
    A. place a bandage and continue working.
    B. wash hands and use antibiotic ointment.
    C. wash hands and inform the doctor.
    D. check the patient's medical history.

Infection Control

45. OSHA requires office personnel to get which kind of immunization?
    A. Hepatitis B
    B. Meningitis
    C. Pneumonia
    D. Strep throat

46. Which of the following used items is considered regulated medical waste by OSHA?
    A. Clinic gowns
    B. Sharps
    C. Masks
    D. Exam gloves

47. The most appropriate gloves to clean and process contaminated instruments are
    A. examination gloves.
    B. overgloves.
    C. sterile gloves.
    D. utility gloves.

48. Chemicals that are identified as a health hazard are color coded
    A. blue.
    B. red.
    C. yellow.
    D. white.

49. When recapping a needle, which of the following techniques should be used?
    A. Two-handed scoop method
    B. One-handed scoop method
    C. Bent needle technique
    D. Broken needle technique

50. The current OSHA standard for exposure to mercury vapor is 0.1 mg/m^3 of air averaged over
    A. 24 hours.
    B. an 8-hour work shift.
    C. a 40-hour work week.
    D. 3 consecutive work days.

51. If a dental office fails to meet safety requirements identified in the OSHA standards, which of the following will result?
    A. OSHA will close the office until the problem is corrected.
    B. OSHA will revoke the dentist's license to practice dentistry.
    C. OSHA will revoke the license and certificates of each dental staff involved.
    D. OSHA will send an inspector to the office on a daily basis.

See p. 71 for the correct answers and rationales

ANSWERS AND RATIONALES:
Infection Control

Patient and Dental Healthcare Worker Education

1. Which airborne infectious disease is a leading cause of death worldwide and is an occupational risk for healthcare workers?

   D. Tuberculosis. Tuberculosis is a bacterial infection of the lungs caused by the *Mycobacterium tuberculosis* bacterium.

2. A pandemic disease is one that

   C. occurs over a large geographic area. A pandemic disease occurs over a large geographic area and may even occur worldwide.

3. Which type of hepatitis is spread through the fecal-oral route?

   A. Hepatitis A. Hepatitis B, C, and D are bloodborne diseases.

4. Dental employers are required to maintain accurate medical records on their employees who are at risk for contamination from bloodborne pathogens. These records are to be kept

   D. the length of employment plus 30 years. Employee medical records are covered under OSHA standards and are required to be kept 30 years beyond the last day of employment.

5. Which of the following items is classified as semicritical?

   D. Rubber dam forceps. Plastic-handled brushes, high-volume evacuator (HVE) tips, rubber dam forceps, X-ray film holders, and amalgam carriers are semicritical instruments.

Standard Precautions to Prevent Disease Transmission

Prevent Cross-Contamination and Transmission

6. Which of the following OSHA standards is written to protect dental healthcare workers from occupational exposure to infectious diseases?

   C. Bloodborne Pathogen Standard. OSHA's Bloodborne Pathogen Standard outlines the precautions taken to protect dental healthcare workers potentially exposed to infectious bodily fluids. Universal/standard precautions and an exposure control plan are a part of the Bloodborne Pathogen Standard.

Infection Control

7. To maintain high filterability, a face mask that is moist from exhaled air should be replaced

    A. every 20 minutes. When a face mask becomes wet, it should be replaced every 20 minutes to maintain its high filterability.

8. Which of the following personal protective barriers should ALWAYS be put on last?

    A. Gloves. The sequence (first to last) in which personal protective barriers should be put on prior to patient treatment is protective clothing, mask, protective eyewear, and gloves.

9. Which of the following is NOT recommended for use as a surface barrier?

    B. Paper tray liners. Surface barriers must be resistant to fluids. Paper products, such as paper tray liners, should not be used as a surface barrier because they are not fluid resistant.

10. Gloves contaminated during dental procedures should be discarded in the

    A. regular waste receptacle. Unless gloves are dripping wet with blood or saliva, they can be routinely disposed of by placing them in the regular waste receptacle.

11. An alcohol-based hand rub should be used only

    C. if there is no visible soil on the hands. Alcohol-based hand rub agents should only be used when there is no visible soil present on the hands. The alcohol in the product kills infectious organisms and then quickly evaporates.

12. Personal protective equipment includes all of the following EXCEPT:

    C. gowns laundered at home. Personal protective equipment (PPE) includes barriers to protect the dental assistant from occupational exposure to potentially infectious splash and splatter. Safety glasses, masks, gloves, and gowns are all PPE; however, gowns worn in the treatment setting should be laundered at the office or sent to commercial cleaners, never at home.

13. Which of the following is NOT true regarding the use of overgloves?

    A. They are acceptable alone as a hand barrier for intraoral procedures. Overgloves are not medical-quality gloves and are not acceptable alone as a hand barrier or for intraoral procedures.

14. Which of the following is the BEST way to clean the high-speed handpiece after patient treatment?

    B. Sterilize in packaging materials. Handpieces are considered critical items due to their ability to penetrate tissue and must be sterilized after each use.

15. When performing a thorough hand washing before gloving, you should rinse your hands with water at what temperature?

    A. Cool. Following washing, the hands should be rinsed with cool water because cool water closes the pores.

Maintain Aseptic Conditions

16. The front desk and walls of the dental office are classified as housekeeping surfaces and should be cleaned with a

    A. low-level disinfectant. There is no evidence that housekeeping surfaces pose a risk to patient contamination, so they should be cleaned periodically with soap and warm water or a low-level disinfectant.

17. To ensure sterilization, steam sterilizers should be loaded so that

    C. instrument packages are packed loosely into the autoclave. Loosely packing the autoclave will allow steam to access all package surfaces to ensure sterilization.

18. Dental instruments that are used in the mouth but do not penetrate tissue or bone are

    B. semicritical instruments. Semicritical instruments are those instruments that are used in the mouth and touch mucous membranes, but do not penetrate soft tissue or bone. Examples would include the mouth mirror, impression trays, and amalgam condenser.

19. Improperly cleaning a dental unit after a procedure could lead to what route of cross-contamination?

    C. Patient to patient. If the dental unit, instruments, handpieces, and attachments are not properly processed after contamination, the opportunity for patient-to-patient transfer increases.

20. Which of the following types of waste must be identified with a biohazard label?

    C. Regulated waste. Infectious waste is regulated waste—it is required to be labeled with the biohazard label and it is never disposed of as general waste.

Perform Sterilization Procedures

21. When evaluating the effectiveness of the sterilizer, what is used as the test medium?

    C. Bacterial endospore. The bacterial endospore is the hardest microorganism to kill and is used as the test standard.

22. After being used for patient treatment and before being sterilized, dental instruments should be

    D. placed in the ultrasonic unit or instrument washer. Ultrasonic cleaners and instrument washers use special cleaners to remove bioburden from contaminated instruments.

23. One of the most common liquid sterilants is

    A. glutaraldehyde. Liquid chemical sterilant/high-level disinfectants used in dental offices include glutaraldehyde, glutaraldehyde-phenate, special hydrogen peroxide, and hydrogen peroxide-peracetic acid. These are used for instruments that would be damaged by heat sterilization.

24. Which method of sterilization is used for instruments that are subject to corrosion?

    A. Dry heat sterilization. Corrosion is caused by moisture. Because dry heat sterilization does not produce moisture, this makes it ideal for dental instruments with moving parts such as orthodontic pliers.

Infection Control

25. Sterilization is defined as

   B. the destruction of all life forms. Sterilization is the destruction of all microorganisms, including spores, and is the standard infection control protocol for dental instruments and handpieces.

26. What is the main disadvantage of a chemical vapor sterilizer?

   C. It must be placed in a well-ventilated area. Chemical vapor sterilizers can cause eye irritation when vented. The chemicals also have a strong unpleasant odor. Good ventilation is essential.

27. Which of the following is the BEST method of preparing instrument packs for the steam autoclave sterilizer?

   C. FDA-approved packaging materials. Sterilization packaging materials are approved by the FDA as medical devices.

28. When the color indicator on the sterilization package changes color after processing, this indicates that the sterilizer

   C. reached the correct temperature. Color indicators on bags, strips, and tape show that, at some point, the sterilizer reached the designated temperature. It does not mean that the optimum time was met or that instruments are sterile.

Environmental Asepsis

29. A good way to reduce cross-contamination of dental materials is to use

   B. disposable materials. Cross-contamination of dental materials could occur during patient care when multiple-dose containers are used. Many of the materials used today come in single-dose packaging to help reduce cross-contamination.

30. Any time a chemical is dispensed into a nonoriginal container, that container should be

   A. marked with a secondary label. Secondary labeling of a material that has been transferred into another container is essential to product identification. Information from the MSDS should be included on the secondary label in case of an accident or emergency.

31. How long should dental impressions be sterilized before the impression is poured?

   B. 15 minutes. Once removed from the patient's mouth, a dental impression should be soaked in a disinfecting solution for 15 minutes prior to pouring in plaster.

32. The best way to minimize cross-contamination of X-ray equipment is to

   C. cover the control panel with plastic. Control panels, knobs, and buttons often have different shapes and designs. It is best to cover these items with plastic to prevent cross-contamination.

33. Which of the following chemicals is a high-level disinfectant?

   B. Chlorine dioxide. Chlorine dioxide is a high-level disinfectant and sterilant. It can be used as a rapid-acting surface disinfectant (3 minutes of contact) or a slower-acting sterilant (6 hours of contact).

34. The active ingredient in chlorine compounds used in dentistry for intermediate-level surface disinfection is

    D. sodium hypochlorite. Chlorine compounds used as intermediate-level surface disinfectants in dentistry contain either sodium hypochlorite or chlorine dioxide as the active ingredient.

35. Which of the following is the best description of an intermediate-level disinfectant?

    C. kills some tuberculosis spores and some viruses. An intermediate-level disinfectant kills some but not all *M. tuberculosis* spores and some viruses.

36. Which of the following solutions is best for cleaning the dental suction lines?

    B. nondetergent, enzymatic cleaning solution. Dental suction lines require proper cleaning to prevent clogging. Use of a nondetergent, enzymatic vacuum cleaning solution will not cause suds and the enzymes will break down the proteins in blood and saliva.

Occupational Safety in the Dental Office

37. What should you use to remove needles from reusable syringes?

    A. Hemostat. To prevent occupational needlestick, the only safe method of removing a needle is with a hemostat or a special instrument designed for that purpose.

38. By law, who provides material safety data sheets for the office?

    B. Manufacturer. Even though the dental practice may receive the MSDSs from the dental vendor, the law requires the manufacturer to generate this document.

39. It is important for the dental assistant to have a foundation in microbiology in order to

    B. prevent disease transmission in the dental setting. The study of microbiology is important for the dental assistant so that he or she will understand the nature of pathogens and understand how to prevent disease transmission in the dental office.

40. The purpose of the Occupational Safety and Health Administration is to protect whom?

    B. Employees. OSHA's primary goal is the health and safety of employees in any occupation.

41. Utilizing universal/standard precautions is enforced by the

    D. OSHA. OSHA is responsible for writing and enforcing standards for employee safety. Universal precautions fall under OSHA's jurisdiction.

42. Which agent is NOT recommended by the CDC for surface disinfection?

    B. Ethyl alcohol. Alcohols evaporate quickly. It would be difficult to keep a surface wet long enough with ethyl alcohol in order to be successful.

Infection Control

43. An office exposure control program must be updated

   C. annually. An exposure control plan must be updated annually and a copy made accessible to all employees.

44. If an employee is stuck with a needle or contaminated instrument, the employee should remove his/her gloves then

   C. wash hands and inform the doctor. If an employee is stuck with a contaminated instrument, he/she should stop working, remove gloves, squeeze the area gently to make it bleed, and wash with an antimicrobial soap. The doctor and/or exposure control officer should be informed and an accident report filed.

45. OSHA requires office personnel to get which kind of immunization?

   A. Hepatitis B. According to OSHA, all employees must be offered the hepatitis B vaccination within 10 days of starting employment.

46. Which of the following used items is considered regulated medical waste by OSHA?

   B. Sharps. Any materials that require special handling in order to dispose of are considered regulated medical waste, including sharps.

47. The most appropriate gloves to clean and process contaminated instruments are

   D. utility gloves. Utility gloves are heavy, thick gloves that provide more physical protection than either sterile gloves or examination gloves and should always be used when contaminated instruments are being cleaned to avoid occupational exposure.

48. Chemicals that are identified as a health hazard are color coded

   A. blue. Blue is given to materials that, upon a very short exposure, could cause death or injury requiring medical attention.

49. When recapping a needle, which of the following techniques should be used?

   B. one-handed scoop method. A one-handed scoop method or the use of a resheathing device is recommended to avoid accidental needlesticks.

50. The current OSHA standard for exposure to mercury vapor is 0.1 mg/m^3 of air averaged over

   A. 24 hours. The National Institute for Occupational Safety and Health is recommending that this be changed to 0.05 mg/m^3 averaged over an 8-hour work shift over a 40-hour work week but, to date, OSHA has not adopted this recommendation.

51. If a dental office fails to meet safety requirements identified in the OSHA standards, which of the following will result?

   A. OSHA will close the office until the problem is corrected. When a dental office fails to meet the safety requirements, a citation may be issued for each violation identified by OSHA. Citations typically result in a fine. When and if the office fails to correct the unsafe issues/conditions, OSHA has the legal authority to close the office until the problem(s) are corrected.

part III

GENERAL CHAIRSIDE (GC)
Practice Exam–1 ½ hours testing time

Directions: Choose the response that best answers each of the following questions.

1. A vasoconstrictor is added to a local anesthetic because it
   A. increases the amount of the local anesthetic given.
   B. minimizes the potential for an allergic reaction.
   C. lengthens the duration of action of the local anesthetic.
   D. decreases the patient's blood pressure.

2. Which of the following may increase the risk of prolonged bleeding for patients?
   A. NSAIDs
   B. Antibiotics
   C. Aspirin
   D. Vitamins

3. Which cement is exothermic and must be mixed on a glass slab?
   A. Glass ionomer
   B. Zinc-oxide eugenol
   C. Polycarboxylate
   D. Zinc phosphate

4. Glass ionomer cement differs from other cements in the unique property of
   A. setting quickly.
   B. releasing fluoride.
   C. being hydrophilic.
   D. stimulating secondary dentin.

5. After receiving a gel or foam fluoride treatment, how long should a patient wait before eating or drinking?
   A. 5 minutes
   B. 10 minutes
   C. 30 minutes
   D. 60 minutes

6. When assembled and positioned properly, the smaller circumference of the matrix band should face which surface of the tooth?
    A. Buccal
    B. Cervical
    C. Occlusal
    D. Lingual

7. Who has legal ownership of all patient records and radiographs?
    A. Dentist
    B. Patient
    C. OSHA
    D. ADA

8. Following the removal of orthodontic brackets, which handpiece is used to remove the bonding material from the tooth?
    A. High-speed
    B. Ultrasonic
    C. Air polisher
    D. Air abrasion

9. An indicator that the final setting time of dental stone has been reached is that the model will be
    A. soft.
    B. hard.
    C. warm and damp.
    D. cool and dry.

10. A patient suffering from hypoglycemia may exhibit which symptom?
    A. Acetone breath
    B. Excessive urination
    C. Excessive thirst
    D. Perspiration

11. The purpose of inverting the dental dam is to
    A. allow the patient the ability to swallow.
    B. allow the dental dam to be removed more easily.
    C. provide increased clamp retention.
    D. prevent salivary leakage.

12. Upon completion of an amalgam restoration, excess amalgam should be disposed of in
    A. the general waste.
    B. a biohazard bag.
    C. a closed container.
    D. the sharps container.

13. An advantage of a diamond bur compared to other dental burs is its
    A. lower cost.
    B. superior cutting edge.
    C. long shank.
    D. longevity.

14. A deficiency in which of the following vitamins may contribute to night blindness?
    A. Vitamin A
    B. Vitamin B
    C. Vitamin C
    D. Vitamin D

15. Which of the following teeth has two roots?
    A. Mandibular first premolar
    B. Mandibular second premolar
    C. Maxillary first premolar
    D. Maxillary second premolar

16. The purpose of attaching a ligature to a dental dam clamp is to
    A. remove the clamp once the procedure is completed.
    B. retrieve the clamp if it becomes dislodged and swallowed.
    C. attach the clamp to the dental dam frame.
    D. attach the clamp to the rubber dam.

17. Patients requiring oral prophylactic antibiotics prior to a procedure should administer the recommended dose at what time?
    A. 30 to 60 minutes after the procedure
    B. 30 to 60 minutes prior to the procedure
    C. 2 hours prior to the procedure
    D. 3 hours prior to the procedure

18. The injection technique most preferred by dentists on the mandibular arch is
    A. local mandibular infiltration.
    B. inferior alveolar nerve block.
    C. periodontal ligamentary injection.
    D. mandibular osseous injection.

19. Which of the following gypsum products has the highest water-to-powder ratio and is the weakest product?
    A. Type I: impression plaster
    B. Type II: model plaster
    C. Type III: laboratory stone
    D. Type IV: orthodontic stone

20. Aspiration allows the dentist to determine the
    A. correct placement of the anesthetic.
    B. effectiveness of the anesthetic.
    C. amount of anesthetic given to the patient.
    D. likelihood that paresthesia will occur.

21. Which of the following is the proper way to make a correction on a patient's chart?
    A. Erase the information and record the new information.
    B. Use white-out and record the new information over the white-out.
    C. Place a single line through the incorrect information and enter the new information on the next line.
    D. Destroy the chart and start a new one.

22. Which type of anesthesia is frequently used on mandibular teeth and injected near a major nerve in order to numb the entire area served by that nerve branch?
    A. Block
    B. Infiltration
    C. Innervation
    D. Induction

23. Which of the following nutrients plays a major role in the development of caries?
    A. Sodium
    B. Proteins
    C. Fats
    D. Carbohydrates

24. The purpose of applying a topical anesthetic prior to an injection is to
    A. reduce postoperative swelling.
    B. prevent infection.
    C. desensitize the area.
    D. increase the effectiveness of the local anesthetic.

25. The examination technique that involves the operator using fingers and hands to evaluate hard and soft tissue is called
    A. probing.
    B. palpation.
    C. instrumentation.
    D. detection.

26. What accessory is required to attach an abrasive disc to a handpiece?
    A. Contra angle
    B. Straight attachment
    C. Nose cone
    D. Mandrel

27. Which of the following dental materials can be used as a desensitizer?
    A. Amalgam
    B. Composite resin
    C. Fluoride
    D. Zinc phosphate

28. Treatment for accidental fluoride overdose includes giving the patient
    A. sodium bicarbonate.
    B. water.
    C. milk.
    D. epinephrine.

29. When dry, a properly etched enamel surface will appear
    A. pitted.
    B. chalky.
    C. glossy.
    D. dark.

30. What is the primary advantage of adding base metals to noble metals in gold-noble alloys?
    A. Decreased cost
    B. Increased resistance to wear
    C. Decreased casting times
    D. Increased esthetics

31. Class II restorations are found on
    A. anterior teeth.
    B. posterior teeth.
    C. canines.
    D. incisors.

32. Which method of toothbrushing emphasizes placing the bristles at a 45-degree angle in the sulcus?
    A. Stillman
    B. Modified Stillman
    C. Charters
    D. Bass

33. Decay located in the pits and fissures of the occlusal surfaces of molars and premolars are considered which classification of caries?
    A. Class I
    B. Class II
    C. Class III
    D. Class IV

34. The material of choice for Class III and Class IV restorations is
    A. composite resin.
    B. amalgam.
    C. glass ionomer.
    D. ceramic.

35. Which of the following is the most appropriate indication for the application of dental sealants?
    A. Anterior teeth with no restorations
    B. Posterior teeth with deep carious lesions
    C. Posterior teeth with pits and fissures
    D. Anterior teeth with shallow pits and fissures

36. Protective bases can be used to prevent
    A. premature contact on the restorative material.
    B. occlusal trauma.
    C. postoperative sensitivity and damage to the pulp.
    D. premature loss of the restorative material.

37. The purpose of retention pins in restorations is to
    A. replace missing cusps.
    B. support core build-ups.
    C. hold crowns and bridges in place.
    D. fill the root canal space.

38. Initial patient contact begins when
    A. the patient is referred to the office for treatment.
    B. the patient calls for a new patient appointment.
    C. the patient arrives at the office for the first time.
    D. the dentist does the comprehensive exam.

39. The significance of the smear layer in restorative dentistry is to
    A. increase bonding strength.
    B. decrease bonding strength.
    C. increase dentinal hypersensitivity.
    D. decrease dentinal hypersensitivity.

40. Chronic overexposure to low concentrations of fluoride in children younger than 6 years of age will most likely cause which of the following conditions?
    A. Acute fluoride poisoning
    B. Anaphylaxis
    C. Decalcification
    D. Dental fluorosis

41. A good way to keep the mouth mirror from fogging while the operator is working is to
    A. blow some air on it.
    B. spray water on it.
    C. soak it in warm water.
    D. wipe it with alcohol.

42. Using the Universal Numbering System, the maxillary right second premolar is designated tooth number
    A. 4.
    B. 5.
    C. 12.
    D. 13.

43. Treatment of alveolitis includes
    A. placement of a periodontal dressing.
    B. placement of sutures.
    C. irrigation with a saline solution.
    D. irrigation with a fluoride solution.

44. Calcium hydroxide can be used for all of the following purposes EXCEPT as a
    A. temporary dental cement.
    B. dental base.
    C. temporary restorative material.
    D. dental varnish.

45. When assisting a right-handed dentist, the dental assistant would use the right hand for
    A. transfer of the air-water syringe.
    B. transfer of hand instruments.
    C. operating a handpiece.
    D. operating the high-volume evacuator.

46. A rapid change in body position, such as when the patient is suddenly placed in the upright position, may result in
    A. partial seizure.
    B. postural hypotension.
    C. apnea.
    D. hyperventilation.

47. When placing the Tofflemire retainer around a tooth, the diagonal slot should face toward the
    A. gingival surface.
    B. occlusal surface.
    C. buccal surface.
    D. lingual surface.

48. What can be used as a visual aid to show the patient the areas in the mouth where debris remains after brushing and flossing?
    A. Dental mirror
    B. Disclosing agent
    C. Diagram of the mouth
    D. Dental floss

49. To prevent the patient from accidentally swallowing the rubber dam clamp, affix
    A. the dental dam before applying the clamp.
    B. a lubricant to the dental dam.
    C. a dental dam napkin under the dental dam.
    D. a piece of dental floss around the clamp.

50. On a prescription, the abbreviation q.i.d. means
    A. as needed.
    B. before meals.
    C. twice a day.
    D. four times a day.

51. Which of the following instruments is used to remove caries during a restorative procedure?
    A. Gingival margin trimmer
    B. Round cutting bur
    C. Enamel hatchet
    D. Curette

52. Which of the following materials would be placed into the prepared tooth FIRST for an amalgam restoration?
    A. Copal resin
    B. Glass ionomer cement
    C. Amalgam
    D. Calcium hydroxide

53. If the dentist is running behind schedule, patients that are waiting for their appointment should be
    A. rescheduled for another day.
    B. offered something to drink.
    C. informed of the situation.
    D. left to wait until called.

54. The cementum, alveolar bone, and gingiva are part of the
    A. enamel.
    B. dentin.
    C. oral mucosa.
    D. periodontium.

55. Antihistamines are used for treating
    A. hypertension.
    B. bacterial endocarditis.
    C. allergic reactions.
    D. apnea.

56. Bitewing radiographs show that there is decay under an existing restoration. This type of caries is called
    A. rampant caries.
    B. recurrent caries.
    C. incipient caries.
    D. root caries.

57. Varnishes are commonly used in amalgam cavity preparations to
    A. seal and protect the dentin from migration of agents into the tooth.
    B. neutralize the acidic pH of the cement base prior to its final setting.
    C. stimulate the formation of reparative dentin in deep cavity preparations.
    D. prevent thermal conductivity.

58. When teaching toothbrushing, the emphasis should be on brushing
    A. at least once a day.
    B. three times a day.
    C. before bedtime.
    D. until complete removal of plaque regardless of time.

59. During an amalgam restoration procedure, articulating paper is used to evaluate the
    A. severity of overbite.
    B. interproximal contacts.
    C. occlusion after carving.
    D. margins of the restoration.

60. If all of the normal treatments for angina do not relieve the pain that the patient is experiencing, the dental team should assume that the patient is suffering from
    A. myocardial infarction.
    B. cardiac arrest.
    C. cardiovascular accident.
    D. heart failure.

61. What is used during a crown and bridge preparation to displace the gingival tissue?
    A. Cotton roll
    B. Retraction cord
    C. Explorer
    D. Rubber dam
    E. Tofflemire matrix band

62. Which of the following may be seen in a patient with bulimia?
    A. Abnormal wear on the occlusal surfaces of the teeth
    B. Abrasion of the tooth enamel
    C. Erosion of the lingual surfaces of the teeth
    D. Dry, cracked tongue

63. After spraying an impression with disinfectant, the impression should be
    A. kept in a warm, dark environment.
    B. sealed in a plastic bag.
    C. rinsed with water and allowed to air dry.
    D. rinsed, then autoclaved.

64. Antibiotic premedication is recommended for patients who may be susceptible for
    A. developing a virus.
    B. developing infective endocarditis.
    C. experiencing extreme anxiety.
    D. experiencing an allergic reaction.

65. Which of the following conditions may occur if excess cement is not removed from the cervical margin after cementation of a crown?
    A. Fracture of the cervical margin of the preparation
    B. Increased occurrence of subgingival caries
    C. Inflammation of interdental papilla
    D. Lateral movement of the adjacent tooth

66. The surgical instrument used to trim alveolar bone and eliminate sharp bony projections is a
    A. curette.
    B. rasp.
    C. rongeur.
    D. hemostat.

67. Xerostomia refers to
    A. dryness of the mouth.
    B. abnormal shortness of the frenum of the tongue.
    C. partial dislocation of the jaw.
    D. a tooth that is below the line of occlusion.

68. A veneer is applied to which surface of a prepared tooth?
    A. Incisal
    B. Facial
    C. Mesial
    D. Distal

69. The primary dentition contains how many premolars?
    A. 0
    B. 2
    C. 4
    D. 8

70. When placing dental cement for a crown or veneer, the assistant should coat the
    A. tooth preparation with a thin layer of material.
    B. tooth preparation with a thick layer of material.
    C. restoration with a thin layer of material.
    D. restoration with a thick layer of material.

71. Which of the following instruments is used to carve the interproximal portion of an amalgam restoration?
    A. Beaver-tail burnisher
    B. Discoid cleoid
    C. Explorer
    D. Hollenback
    E. Woodson

72. Which of the following is part of a full maxillary denture?
    A. Framework
    B. Post dam
    C. Rest
    D. Connector

73. What is the treatment for angina pectoris?
    A. Acetaminophen
    B. Dextrose
    C. Epinephrine
    D. Nitroglycerin

74. What is used to determine the color of the composite resin material during the restorative procedure?
    A. Transilluminator
    B. Natural light
    C. Vitalometer
    D. Scanner
    E. Shade guide

75. Which filler type of composite resin has the strongest makeup and is used commonly for posterior restorations?
    A. Autofilled
    B. Macrofilled
    C. Microfilled
    D. Nanofilled
    E. Hybrid

76. The goal of water fluoridation is to adjust the fluoride content to
    A. 0.2 ppm.
    B. 0.4 ppm.
    C. 1.0 ppm.
    D. 2.0 ppm.

77. All of the following instruments are required for packing retraction cord EXCEPT for
    A. a mirror.
    B. cotton pliers.
    C. a discoid cleoid.
    D. an explorer.

Refer to the dental chart illustrated below for questions 78 to 82.

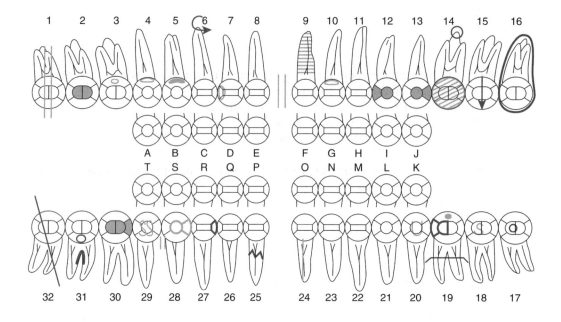

78. The charting symbol illustrated between tooth number 28 and tooth number 29 designates
    A. hypersensitivity.
    B. mobility.
    C. open contact.
    D. overhang.

79. The charting symbol illustrated on tooth number 24 indicates
    A. mobility.
    B. fractured root.
    C. pontic.
    D. root canal.

80. Which of the following conditions exist between tooth number 8 and tooth number 9?
    A. Supernumerary tooth
    B. Overhang
    C. Diastema
    D. Food impaction

81. Which of the following restorations is charted on tooth number 29?
    A. Sealant
    B. Stainless steel crown
    C. Temporary acrylic crown
    D. Full gold crown

82. Which of the following conditions exists on the permanent maxillary left central incisor?
    A. Veneer
    B. Pontic
    C. Fractured root
    D. Implant

83. Which of the following actions should be taken first in managing an office emergency?
    A. Calling for EMS
    B. Performing basic life support
    C. Performing CPR
    D. Sustaining life

84. During a composite procedure, sectional matrices are used in conjunction with which of the following?
    A. Tofflemire retainer
    B. Tension ring
    C. Celluloid clip
    D. Cervical clamp

85. The primary objective of amalgam polishing is to
    A. improve cosmetic appearance.
    B. reduce the chance of galvanic shock.
    C. create a smoother surface with fewer irregularities.
    D. remove excess mercury from the surface of the filling.

86. An accurate record of a patient's financial history with the dental office should be recorded
    A. in the patient's progress notes.
    B. on a manual or electronic ledger card.
    C. on the patient's walk-out statement.
    D. with the accountant for tax records.

87. Topical anesthetic is applied prior to giving an injection in order to
    A. act as an antiseptic.
    B. prevent infection.
    C. reduce bleeding at the injection site.
    D. desensitize the tissue at the injection site.

88. In an emergency, check the patient for a pulse at which artery?
    A. Brachial
    B. Femoral
    C. Radial
    D. Carotid

89. If a right-handed operator is preparing tooth number 3 for a crown, the dental assistant would place the bevel of the high-velocity evacuator
    A. parallel to the buccal surface of the tooth being prepared.
    B. parallel to the lingual surface of the tooth being prepared.
    C. distal to the left maxillary tuberosity from the buccal side.
    D. distal to the left maxillary tuberosity from the lingual side.

90. The primary cause of syncope (fainting) in the dental office is
    A. allergic reaction to local anesthetic.
    B. toxic reaction to local anesthetic.
    C. dental anxiety.
    D. length of dental procedure.

91. During an amalgam procedure, which instrument is used to pack the amalgam firmly into the tooth preparation?
    A. Amalgam carrier
    B. Condenser
    C. Ball burnisher
    D. Excavator

92. Which of the following is associated with the intake of sugar-free sodas and dental caries?
    A. A decrease in saliva production
    B. An increase in saliva production
    C. A decrease in acidity
    D. An increase in acidity

93. The properly seated dental assistant is
    A. on the same plane as the dentist.
    B. 2 to 4 in above the dentist.
    C. 4 to 6 in above the dentist.
    D. 6 to 8 in above the dentist.

94. Calcium hydroxide is used under new restorations to
    A. reduce thermal sensitivity.
    B. reduce marginal leakage.
    C. seal dentinal tubules.
    D. stimulate reparative dentin.

95. Subgingival calculus is removed using a
    A. curette.
    B. chisel.
    C. sickle.
    D. hoe.

96. Impressions should be disinfected
    A. at the dental lab check-in.
    B. at the chairside upon removal.
    C. before rinsing with water.
    D. for an hour before pouring in gypsum.

97. Which of the following choices represents the lowest ratio, meaning greatest concentration, of vaso-constrictor in local anesthetic?
    A. 1:20,000
    B. 1:50,000
    C. 1:100,000
    D. 1:200,000

98. The attachments at the sides of a three-unit bridge are called
    A. pontics.
    B. abutments.
    C. anchors.
    D. spacers.

99. Which of the following refers to an allergic response that could threaten a patient's life?
    A. Grand mal
    B. Myocardial infarction
    C. Anaphylaxis
    D. Hypersensitivity

100. A patient with dental insurance is classified as the
    A. primary.
    B. provider.
    C. subscriber.
    D. carrier.

101. The portion of the bridge that replaces the missing tooth is the
    A. pontic.
    B. abutment.
    C. anchor.
    D. spacer.

102. To minimize a patient's gag reflex while taking a maxillary alginate impression, the dental assistant would use
    A. cold water and calcium sulfate.
    B. hot water and fast-set material.
    C. less material than normal.
    D. a tray that is one size smaller than the patient's arch size.

103. The operator has prepared an MO amalgam preparation on tooth number 3. The interproximal box is rough and needs to be smoothed. What would you pass to the operator?
    A. Spoon excavator
    B. Round bur
    C. Interproximal carver
    D. Enamel hatchet

104. When should sealants be placed on a tooth?
    A. Right before the tooth has fully erupted
    B. As soon as the tooth has fully erupted
    C. Six months after eruption is complete
    D. After premolars form

105. During an operative procedure, the best way to keep the tooth from overheating and damaging the pulp is to
    A. place a liner prior to the procedure to act as an insulator.
    B. spray a mixture of air and water over the tooth.
    C. suction constantly during the prep phase to remove heat.
    D. spray air only over the tooth to remove heat.

106. A patient who begins to breathe deeply and rapidly is experiencing
    A. hypoventilation.
    B. hyperventilation.
    C. apnea.
    D. bradypnea.

107. Which wall of the cavity preparation is perpendicular to the long axis of the tooth?
    A. Axial wall
    B. Interface wall
    C. Proximal wall
    D. Pulpal wall

108. Which classification of restoration does NOT require a matrix band?
    A. I
    B. II
    C. III
    D. IV

109. When punching a rubber dam for a restorative procedure, the anchor tooth should be
    A. the tooth being prepared.
    B. the tooth that is ligated.
    C. 1 or 2 teeth to the distal.
    D. 1 or 2 teeth to the mesial.

110. During an emergency, the AED is used to provide which of the following to the heart?
    A. Oxygen
    B. Lower blood pressure
    C. Electricity
    D. Epinephrine

111. The agents that provide a temporary numbing effect on nerve endings located on the surface of the oral mucosa are
    A. local anesthetics.
    B. topical anesthetics.
    C. general anesthetics.
    D. inhalation anesthetics.

112. Mrs. Applebee recently had an MOD amalgam placed in tooth number 14. Her tooth was temperature sensitive for about a week and then the sensitivity subsided. This temporary hypersensitivity was most likely due to which of the following?
    A. Chronic pulpitis
    B. Pulpal hyperemia
    C. Traumatic occlusion
    D. Galvanic shock

113. What is achieved by injecting the anesthetic solution directly into the tissue at the site of the dental procedure?
    A. Block anesthesia
    B. Inferior alveolar nerve block anesthesia
    C. Infiltration anesthesia
    D. Incisive nerve block

114. Anaphylaxis is considered to be
    A. a mild allergic reaction.
    B. a life-threatening allergic reaction.
    C. a severe asthma attack.
    D. a petit mal seizure.

115. During the finishing of a Class III composite restoration, which of the following instruments may be used to remove excess flash and to smooth the interproximal area?
    A. Abrasive strip
    B. Mounted polishing disc
    C. Sand paper disc
    D. #7404 egg carbide finishing bur

116. Hardness of a material is ranked using the
    A. Richter scale.
    B. Mercalli scale.
    C. Mohs scale.
    D. Heimlich scale.

117. Which of the following instruments are NOT used in refining and finishing the cavity walls and margins of the cavity preparation?
    A. Enamel hatchets
    B. Margin trimmers
    C. Fissure bur in a high-speed handpiece
    D. Spoon excavators

118. When a patient fails to show for an appointment, the scheduling assistant should
    A. call the patient and summarize the conversation in the patient's chart.
    B. inactivate the patient's file until the patient calls for another appointment.
    C. leave a message on the patient's voicemail asking why the appointment was missed.
    D. send the patient a bill for the missed appointment.

119. In four-handed dentistry, the area of exchange is located
    A. across the chest near the patient's chin.
    B. across the stomach area.
    C. behind the patient's head.
    D. over the patient's mouth.

120. The dental team member most likely to be in charge of calling the emergency medical services is the
    A. business assistant.
    B. dentist.
    C. chairside assistant.
    D. roving assistant.

See p. 117 for the correct answers and rationales.

RADIATION HEALTH AND SAFETY (RHS)
Practice Exam–1¼ hours testing time

Directions: Choose the response that best answers each of the following questions.

1. Which of the following film speeds is the fastest?
   A. A
   B. D
   C. E
   D. F

2. The purpose of the aluminum filter is to
   A. erase the short wavelengths from the X-ray beam.
   B. diminish the size and shape of the X-ray beam.
   C. allow for a more penetrating primary beam.
   D. reduce the intensity of the primary beam.

3. Overexposure to a safelight will produce a film that is
   A. clear.
   B. fogged.
   C. yellow.
   D. stained.

4. What describes a radiograph's darkness?
   A. Density
   B. Contrast
   C. Milliamperage
   D. Penumbra

5. The maximum permissible dose of radiation for an operator is
   A. 1 REM or 0.01 Sv per year.
   B. 1 REM or 0.05 Sv per year.
   C. 5 REMs or 0.01 Sv per year.
   D. 5 REMs or 0.05 Sv per year.

6. Areas that appear dark on a radiograph are called
   A. radiopaque.
   B. radiolucent.
   C. dense.
   D. intense.

7. Cells with a high reproductive rate are considered to be
   A. radioresistant.
   B. radiosensitive.
   C. radiolucent.
   D. radiopaque.

8. A radiograph that is exposed using a high kVp will have
   A. many shades of gray.
   B. black and white areas only.
   C. a decrease in sharpness.
   D. a decrease in density.

9. Which of the four components of a film packet reduces secondary radiation?
    A. Outer wrap
    B. Black paper
    C. Radiograph film
    D. Lead foil

10. The largest intraoral film size is
    A. #1.
    B. #2.
    C. #3.
    D. #4.

11. Which of the following helps reduce the X-ray exposure of a patient?
    A. Tubehead
    B. Film badge
    C. Collimator
    D. Focusing cup

Refer to the radiographs below for questions 12 to 14.

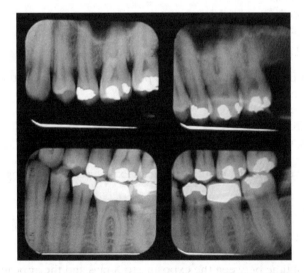

From: Scheid R. *Woelfel's Dental Anatomy: Its Relevance to Dentistry.* Philadelphia: Lippincott Williams & Wilkins; 2007.

12. In the upper left radiograph, the film was positioned too far
    A. apically.
    B. mesially.
    C. distally.
    D. occlusally.

13. The technical error in the upper right radiograph is an example of
    A. elongation.
    B. foreshortening.
    C. reversed film.
    D. bent film.

14. Which technical errors are illustrated in the lower radiographs?
    A. Excessive vertical angulation
    B. Insufficient horizontal angulation
    C. Film placement
    D. Cone cut

15. Which of the following is the major advantage of a panoramic radiograph?
    A. Lower cost to the patient compared to intraoral films
    B. Entire dentition seen on one film
    C. Increased detail compared to intraoral films
    D. Reduced radiation exposure to the thyroid gland

16. Which of the following structures will appear radiopaque on a radiograph?
    A. PFM
    B. Soft tissue
    C. Tooth decay
    D. Dental pulp

17. Which of the following anatomical structures will appear radiolucent on a radiograph?
    A. Nasal septum
    B. Genial tubercles
    C. Mental foramen
    D. Cortical bone

18. Which of the following cells are the MOST radiosensitive?
    A. Muscle cells
    B. Nerve cells
    C. Bone marrow cells
    D. Salivary gland cells

19. The number of waves that pass a given point per unit of time is the
    A. wavelength.
    B. wave height.
    C. wave frequency.
    D. wave crest.

20. If a film is reversed in the mouth during an exposure, the resulting image will look
    A. darker.
    B. lighter.
    C. larger.
    D. smaller.

21. The period of time between the exposure to X-rays and the appearance of radiation damage is called the
    A. recovery period.
    B. latent period.
    C. genetic period.
    D. somatic period.

22. Which of the following conditions can be identified on a radiograph?
    A. Herpetic lesions
    B. Aphthous ulcers
    C. Salivary stones
    D. Frena

23. Which of the following types of ionizing radiation produce the least amount of scatter radiation?
    A. Long wavelength radiation
    B. Short wavelength radiation
    C. Moderate wavelength radiation
    D. Extremely long wavelength radiation

24. How often should automatic processing solutions be changed?
    A. Daily
    B. Every week
    C. Every 3 to 4 weeks
    D. Every 6 months

25. Elongation of an image on a radiograph may be caused by
    A. insufficient vertical angulation.
    B. extended target-film distance.
    C. poor patient positioning.
    D. poor film quality.

26. Regulations state that an X-ray unit operating above 70 kVp must have a total filtration of
    A. 1.0 mm.
    B. 2.0 mm.
    C. 2.5 mm.
    D. 3.5 mm.

27. A radiopaque landmark found superimposed over the apical areas of the molars in the maxilla is the
    A. external oblique ridge.
    B. floor of the sinus.
    C. incisive foramen.
    D. inverted Y.

28. When using the bisecting angle technique, the vertical angulation of the maxillary premolar exposure is
    A. +10.
    B. +25.
    C. +30.
    D. +45.

29. The advantage of using intensifying screens in extraoral radiography is
    A. reduced exposure time.
    B. decreased processing time.
    C. decreased distortion.
    D. increased film contrast.

30. Failure to fix films long enough will result in a radiograph with
    A. white spots.
    B. black lines running through it.
    C. decreased density.
    D. a brown tint.

31. The negatively charged part of the X-ray tube is the
    A. cathode.
    B. anode.
    C. target.
    D. focal spot.

32. What is the best way for an assistant to evaluate the amount of radiation he or she receives?
    A. Test the X-ray machine for leakage.
    B. Go to a physician to check for cell damage.
    C. Wear a film badge everywhere at all times.
    D. Wear a dosimeter at work for 3 months.

Radiation Health and Safety

33. At the patient's skin, the diameter of the X-ray beam should not exceed
    A. 1.25 in.
    B. 2.0 in.
    C. 2.75 in.
    D. 3.35 in.

34. Excessive vertical angulation causes
    A. foreshortened tooth structures.
    B. elongated tooth structures.
    C. overlapping of interproximal areas.
    D. magnification of tooth structures.

35. Which of the following structures will appear the most radiopaque on a radiograph?
    A. Amalgam restoration
    B. Pulp chamber
    C. Paper points
    D. Periodontal ligament

36. If the developer solution is exhausted, the radiograph will be
    A. overdeveloped.
    B. underdeveloped.
    C. clear.
    D. dark.

37. Which of the following is a property of X-rays?
    A. They travel at the speed of sound.
    B. They do not cause biologic changes in cells.
    C. They have no mass or weight.
    D. They have a negative charge.

38. The maximum yearly permissible dose of radiation that a pregnant woman should receive is
    A. 100 mSv (or 10,000 millirem/mrem).
    B. 50 mSv (or 5,000 millirem/mrem).
    C. 5 mSv (or 5,000 millirem/mrem).
    D. 1 mSv (or 1,000 millirem/mrem).

39. What is the minimum distance an operator should stand during an X-ray exposure?
    A. 4 ft
    B. 6 ft
    C. 8 ft
    D. 10 ft

40. Which of the following would the operator adjust in order to increase the quantity of electrons inside the X-ray tube?
    A. Milliamperage
    B. Kilovoltage
    C. Filtration
    D. Target-to-object distance

41. Overexposure of the skin to radiation will cause a redness or sunburned appearance called
    A. contact rash.
    B. dermatitis.
    C. erythema.
    D. edema.

42. What must be done with nondisposable dental film holders after each use?
    A. They must be disinfected with an intermediate level disinfectant.
    B. They must be placed in a high level disinfectant for 30 minutes.
    C. They must be sterilized.
    D. They should never be used.

43. The target in the X-ray tube is composed of what metal?
    A. Copper
    B. Aluminum
    C. Lead
    D. Tungsten

44. Identify the anatomical structure that will appear radiolucent on a radiograph.
    A. Mental foramen
    B. Genial tubercles
    C. Nasal spine
    D. External oblique ridge

45. A collar on a lead apron is used to protect the patient's
    A. vocal cords.
    B. thyroid gland.
    C. spinal cord.
    D. heart and lungs.

46. Overlapping images is caused by
    A. incorrect vertical angulation.
    B. incorrect horizontal angulation.
    C. excessive bending of the film.
    D. placing the film in the mouth backwards.

47. What type of X-rays produce the radiographic image in the form of the latent image?
    A. Remnant
    B. Primary
    C. Secondary
    D. Photoelectric

48. Which of the following is the correct test to detect light leaks in the darkroom?
    A. Reference radiograph test
    B. Coin test
    C. Clearing time test
    D. Fogging test

49. A structure that stops or absorbs X-rays will appear
    A. radiolucent.
    B. radiopaque.
    C. radiographic.
    D. radiosensitive.

50. The most penetrating X-rays have a
    A. low frequency.
    B. long frequency.
    C. short wavelength.
    D. long wavelength.

51. The RINN XCP is assembled to expose a mandibular right molar periapical. Which of the following areas can be exposed without having to reassemble the film holder?
    A. Maxillary right molar
    B. Maxillary left molar
    C. Mandibular left molar
    D. Mandibular anterior

52. On which radiograph would the inverted Y be seen?
    A. Maxillary premolar periapical
    B. Maxillary canine periapical
    C. Mandibular premolar periapical
    D. Mandibular canine periapical

53. ALARA stands for
    A. as long as radiation is absorbed.
    B. adequate levels as reasonably allowed.
    C. as low as reasonably achievable.
    D. a legally allotted radiation amount.

54. A step-wedge is a device used to test the
    A. automatic processor.
    B. film freshness.
    C. safelight strength.
    D. darkroom light leaks.

55. To avoid cone cuts on a radiograph, the operator must
    A. center the PID over the film.
    B. position the central ray to pass thru the interproximal spaces.
    C. use the correct vertical angulation.
    D. use the correct horizontal angulation.

56. Assuming that the mA and kVp stay the same, if the focal-film distance doubles, the exposure time needed to produce a quality film quadruples. This concept is known as
    A. ALARA.
    B. inverse square law.
    C. intensity factor.
    D. step-wedge.

57. When taking a radiographic survey on a child under the age of 10 years, the exposure (mAs) should be reduced by
    A. 15%.
    B. 25%.
    C. 50%.
    D. 75%.

58. Identify the correct setting that would indicate the PID pointing to the floor.
    A. 0
    B. +10
    C. −10
    D. −65

59. Decreasing the amount of time a duplicating film is exposed to light will result in a film that is
    A. darker.
    B. lighter.
    C. clearer.
    D. black.

60. A size #3 film is used for
   A. a periapical radiograph on an adult.
   B. a bitewing radiograph on an adult.
   C. a bitewing radiograph on a child.
   D. an occlusal radiograph on an adult.

61. Which of the following is responsible for the recording of the image on the radiograph?
   A. Gelatin emulsion
   B. Polyester base
   C. Silver halide crystals
   D. Lead backing

62. Which anatomic structure will be present on a mandibular anterior radiograph?
   A. Mental foramen
   B. Incisive foramen
   C. Lingual foramen
   D. Mandibular foramen

63. Bitewing radiographs are most useful in diagnosis of
   A. periapical abscess.
   B. interproximal decay.
   C. impacted teeth.
   D. supernumerary teeth.

64. Bitewing radiographs are used to locate
   A. periodontal disease.
   B. apical lesions.
   C. impacted teeth.
   D. interproximal caries.

65. Patients are protected from radiation by the filter in the tubehead that
   A. adjusts the exposure impulses.
   B. keeps the wavelengths short.
   C. eliminates stronger wavelengths.
   D. absorbs all stray radiation.

66. When processing radiographs manually, the time and temperature for developing is
   A. 3 minutes at 62° F.
   B. 4 minutes at 65° F.
   C. 5 minutes at 68° F.
   D. 6 minutes at 72° F.

67. Film speed is determined by
   A. kilovoltage.
   B. milliamperage.
   C. the size of the crystal.
   D. the size of the film being used.

68. Radiation that impacts future generations has what kind of effect?
   A. Cumulative
   B. Genetic
   C. Somatic
   D. Biologic

69. A correctly placed premolar bitewing will include the
    A. distal of the canine.
    B. distal of the first molar.
    C. distal of the lateral incisor.
    D. mesial of the canine.

70. The mandibular canal is found on which film?
    A. Molar bitewing
    B. Maxillary molar PA
    C. Mandibular central PA
    D. Mandibular molar PA

71. In which exposure would one identify the genial tubercle as a landmark?
    A. Mandibular canine
    B. Mandibular premolar
    C. Mandibular incisor
    D. Maxillary molar

72. The maxillary tuberosity is found on which film?
    A. Maxillary molar
    B. Maxillary incisor
    C. Maxillary premolar
    D. Maxillary canine

73. Which of the following anatomical landmarks is not visible in the mandibular molar exposure?
    A. External oblique ridge
    B. Mental foramen
    C. Mandibular canal
    D. Mylohyoid ridge

74. Compared to ANSI D-speed film, F-speed film
    A. is less sensitive.
    B. requires more radiation.
    C. results in more exposure to the patient.
    D. requires less exposure time.

75. Old developing solutions will cause the films to appear
    A. brown.
    B. dark.
    C. light.
    D. fuzzy.

76. Which of the following can result in a light film?
    A. Exposure to white light
    B. Unsafe safelight
    C. Reversed film
    D. Overdevelopment

77. The process of removing electrons from atoms is called
    A. radiosensitivity.
    B. ionization.
    C. gamma effect.
    D. ultraviolet exposure.

Refer to the radiograph below for questions 78 to 82.

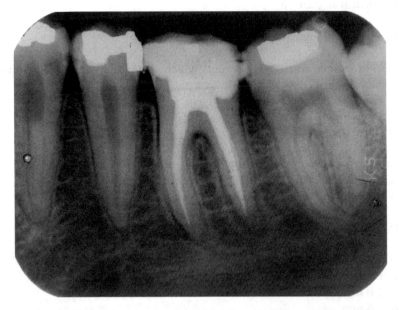

From: Scheid R. *Woelfel's Dental Anatomy: Its Relevance to Dentistry.* Philadelphia: Lippincott Williams & Wilkins; 2007.

78. This radiograph is an example of which of the following?
    A. Bitewing radiograph
    B. Interproximal radiograph
    C. Periapical radiograph

79. What size film was used for this radiographic exposure?
    A. 0
    B. 1
    C. 2
    D. 3

80. The radiopaque areas visible in the mesial and distal roots of the molar are
    A. posts and core.
    B. sedative restorations.
    C. implants.
    D. root canals.

81. The radiopaque material visible in the roots of the mandibular molar is most likely
    A. composite core resin.
    B. gutta percha.
    C. steel points.
    D. titanium pins.

82. The restoration visible in the second premolar is a/an
    A. MO amalgam.
    B. DO gold onlay.
    C. DO amalgam.
    D. DO composite.

83. Which of the following factors determines exposure time?
    A. PID length
    B. Vertical angulation
    C. Size of patient
    D. Horizontal angulation

84. Correct horizontal angulation prevents which of the following radiographic errors?
    A. Elongation
    B. Foreshortening
    C. Overlapping contacts
    D. Blurred image

85. What is the purpose of a risk management program for taking radiographs in the dental office?
    A. Reduce the chance of a malpractice suit
    B. Appease the insurance company
    C. Allow patients a grievance procedure
    D. Get a patient's implied consent

86. An X-ray machine operating at 70 kVp must have how much aluminum filtration in order to comply with federal law?
    A. 1.0 mm
    B. 1.5 mm
    C. 2.0 mm
    D. 2.5 mm

87. Static from improperly handling film will appear to have which pattern on the finished film?
    A. Herringbone
    B. Fuzzy
    C. Lightening
    D. Double

88. The glass wall and insulating oil acts as what type of filtration for X-ray photons generated in the tube-head?
    A. Secondary
    B. Inherent
    C. Primary
    D. Auxiliary

89. The total amount of radiation a dental patient receives
    A. lasts only a few hours.
    B. is not harmful in small doses.
    C. comes from the environment.
    D. is cumulative over a lifetime.

Refer to the radiograph below for questions 90 and 91.

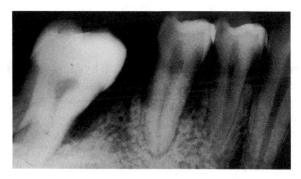

From: Scheid R. *Woelfel's Dental Anatomy: Its Relevance to Dentistry.* Philadelphia: Lippincott Williams & Wilkins; 2007.

90. Which tooth is missing?
    A. Number 2
    B. Number 19
    C. Number 29
    D. Number 30

91. The radiolucent area involving the molar and premolars shows
    A. radicular cysts.
    B. severe bone loss.
    C. normal bone level.
    D. abfraction.

92. Which of the following is one of the earliest clinical signs of overexposure to X-rays?
    A. Malaise
    B. Erythema
    C. Vomiting
    D. Cancer

93. Which of the following is considered to be the yearly maximum permissible dose (MPD) for dental patients?
    A. 0.5 mSv/5 REM
    B. 5 mSv/0.5 REM
    C. 10 mSv/0.1 REM
    D. 50 mSv/5 REM

94. The primary purpose of monitoring X-ray equipment is to
    A. keep track of machine usage.
    B. check for radiation leaks.
    C. track changes in film density.
    D. equally distribute exposure to staff.

95. The primary advantage of an automatic film processor is that
    A. no darkroom is needed.
    B. films are read dry.
    C. films are mounted immediately.
    D. there is no need for chemicals.

96. During X-ray exposure, a thyroid collar should be placed on
    A. children under the age of 12 years.
    B. females.
    C. males.
    D. all patients.

97. Radiation that has been deflected from its path by impact with matter is called
    A. scatter radiation.
    B. primary radiation.
    C. secondary radiation.
    D. stray radiation.

98. Leaving the radiograph in the final water bath too long will cause the image to
    A. lighten.
    B. become clear.
    C. darken.
    D. wrinkle.

Refer to the radiograph below for questions 99 and 100.

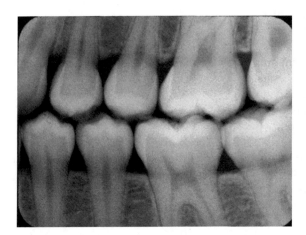

From: Scheid R. *Woelfel's Dental Anatomy: Its Relevance to Dentistry.* Philadelphia: Lippincott Williams & Wilkins; 2007.

99. This radiograph is an example of a
    A. bitewing radiograph.
    B. periapical radiograph.

100. This radiograph illustrates the
    A. left molar.
    B. left premolar.
    C. right premolar.
    D. right molar.

See p. 131 for the correct answers and rationales.

INFECTION CONTROL (ICE)
Practice Exam–1 ¼ hours testing time

Directions: Choose the response that best answers each of the following questions.

1. Vaccination of employees against the hepatitis B virus must be offered within how many days following the start date of employment?
    A. 5 days
    B. 7 days
    C. 10 days
    D. 30 days

2. The MOST effective method of preventing cross-contamination in the dental office is
    A. using an intermediate level disinfectant on all surfaces.
    B. soaking contaminated instruments in a high level disinfectant.
    C. wearing the proper PPE for all procedures.
    D. performing proper handwashing.

3. Which of the following will determine that instrument sterilization was achieved?
    A. Process integrators
    B. Physical monitors
    C. Biological monitors
    D. Chemical indicators

4. A high level disinfectant must have the ability to kill
    A. bacterial spores.
    B. the hepatitis B virus.
    C. tuberculosis.
    D. fungus.

5. Which of the following types of latex allergy is the MOST common?
    A. Irritant allergic reaction
    B. Immediate allergic reaction
    C. Allergic contact dermatitis
    D. Irritant contact dermatitis

6. Biofilm is made up of a thin film of
    A. colonized bacterial cells.
    B. salivary glycoprotein.
    C. calculus.
    D. dietary sugars.

7. Dental instruments that are used in the mouth but do not penetrate tissue or bone are
    A. critical instruments.
    B. semicritical instruments.
    C. noncritical instruments.
    D. nonsterile instruments.

Infection Control

8. Who is responsible for supplying Material Safety Data Sheets to the dental office?
   A. Dentist
   B. Dental assistant
   C. Manufacturer
   D. Distributor

9. Coming into contact with which of the following is MOST likely to cause the spread of herpes in the dental office?
   A. Respiratory secretions
   B. Saliva
   C. Blood
   D. Lesions

10. The main disadvantage to using a dry heat sterilizer is the
    A. ventilation that must be used.
    B. tendency to rust instruments.
    C. long cycle time.
    D. inability to use cassettes.

11. The effects of chronic chemical toxicity include
    A. arthritis.
    B. cancer.
    C. vertigo.
    D. vomiting.

12. Critical items must be treated with which of the following methods to prevent the spread of infection?
    A. Disinfection
    B. Barriers
    C. Sterilization
    D. Sanitation

13. Saliva ejectors and plastic high-volume evacuator tips should be
    A. disposed of after use.
    B. disinfected with a chemical agent.
    C. sterilized in an autoclave.
    D. sterilized in a dry heat sterilizer.

14. An example of an engineering control is
    A. implementing office policies and procedures.
    B. changing the manner of how a task is performed.
    C. isolating or removing a hazard.
    D. mandating that all employees complete annual training.

15. An example of a bloodborne pathogen is
    A. hepatitis A.
    B. hepatitis C.
    C. tuberculosis.
    D. influenza.

16. A positive biological monitoring test result indicates
    A. disinfection was achieved.
    B. sterilization failed.
    C. all spores were destroyed.
    D. the autoclave is functioning properly.

17. Which of the following is considered regulated waste?
    A. Cement mixing pads
    B. Utility gloves
    C. Used anesthetic needles
    D. Used drinking cups

18. Which of the following agencies has the authority to enforce infection control regulations?
    A. Centers for Disease Control and Prevention (CDC)
    B. American Dental Association (ADA)
    C. National Institute for Occupational Safety and Health (NIOSH)
    D. Occupational Safety and Health Administration (OSHA)

19. Destruction of all microorganisms is called
    A. cleaning.
    B. sterilization.
    C. disinfection.
    D. sanitation.

20. A chemical labeled a disinfectant is unable to kill
    A. the HIV virus.
    B. the hepatitis B virus.
    C. the H1N1 virus.
    D. bacterial endospores.

21. According to the OSHA Bloodborne Pathogen Standard, which of the following is prohibited in the dental operatory and sterilization areas?
    A. Carpeting on the floor
    B. Cloth upholstered chairs and stools
    C. Eating and drinking
    D. Pouring up study models

22. The safety and effectiveness of sterilization equipment in the dental office is controlled by the
    A. Environmental Protection Agency.
    B. Occupational Safety and Health Administration.
    C. Centers for Disease Control and Prevention.
    D. Food and Drug Administration.

23. Microorganisms that produce disease in humans are known as
    A. nonpathogens.
    B. pathogens.
    C. microflora.
    D. biofilm.

24. Which of the following tasks would require the dental assisting to wear utility gloves?
    A. Disinfecting the operatory following patient care
    B. Preparing the operatory for patient care
    C. Taking an alginate impression
    D. Retrieving instruments from a drawer during patient care

25. Which intermediate level disinfectant may contribute to staining of clinical surfaces?
    A. Phenolics
    B. Iodophors
    C. Quaternary ammonium compounds
    D. Sodium bromide

26. The agency dedicated to providing educational material to dental health professionals is the
    A. ADA.
    B. CDC.
    C. OSAP.
    D. OSHA.

27. The patient notes on her medical history that she has active tuberculosis. She is scheduled for a crown preparation. How does her condition affect her dental treatment?
    A. She should be treated like any other patient utilizing standard precautions.
    B. She should be treated with double gloves and extra sterilization of the instruments used.
    C. Her treatment should be postponed until her disease is no longer active.
    D. She should be treated with prophylactic premedication before the procedure.

28. To properly dispose of a blood-soaked gauze square, place it in
    A. a regulated trash bag.
    B. the general waste bag.
    C. a leak-proof sharps container.
    D. the sterilizer and then the general waste bag.

29. OSHA requires, which of the following dental employees receive training in the Bloodborne Pathogen Standard?
    A. Dental sales representative
    B. Insurance coordinator
    C. Chairside assistant
    D. Dental lab delivery person

30. Overgloves should be used when
    A. disinfecting the operatory after patient care.
    B. performing an intraoral examination.
    C. preparing the operatory for patient care.
    D. opening a drawer during patient treatment.

31. The major advantage to using liquid chemical sterilization is that
    A. sterilization is achieved in a short period of time.
    B. corrosion or rusting of instruments will not occur.
    C. items that would be damaged by heat can be sterilized using this method.
    D. items do not require the use of pouches or bags.

32. Which of the following conditions would contraindicate the use of nitrous oxide-oxygen conscious sedation?
    A. Anxiety
    B. Heart disease
    C. Nasal obstruction
    D. Kidney disease

33. Sodium hypochlorite is recommended as a disinfectant for
    A. clinical contact surfaces.
    B. housekeeping surfaces.
    C. surfaces covered by barriers.
    D. surfaces that are easily stained by iodophors.

34. Which of the following items should be disinfected before handling in the dental laboratory?
    A. Plaster model
    B. Model articulator
    C. Impression
    D. Implant

35. Which method of sterilization is recommended for items that will be used immediately after removal from the sterilizer?
    A. Dry heat sterilization
    B. Steam sterilization
    C. Flash sterilization
    D. Chemical sterilization

36. What type of water does the ADA and the CDC recommend when performing surgical procedures?
    A. Saline water
    B. Sterile water
    C. Distilled water
    D. Reservoir water

37. What type of immunity occurs when a person receives a vaccination for a disease?
    A. Active natural immunity
    B. Active artificial immunity
    C. Passive natural immunity
    D. Passive artificial immunity

38. Which mode of transmission involves contact with a contaminated instrument or surface?
    A. Airborne transmission
    B. Droplet transmission
    C. Direct contact
    D. Indirect contact

39. Microorganisms that accumulate on wet surfaces, such as on the inside of dental waterline tubing, are called
    A. bioburden.
    B. biofilm.
    C. pathogens.
    D. protozoa.

40. Which of the following diseases is considered a chronic infection?
    A. Influenza
    B. Chickenpox
    C. Hepatitis B carrier state
    D. Strep throat

41. Which of the following agencies would be LEAST concerned with infection control standards?
    A. CDC
    B. FDA
    C. OSAP
    D. NIOSH

42. The MOST effective method of confirming sterilization of instruments is with
    A. chemical indicators.
    B. chemical integrators.
    C. bacterial spore testing.
    D. physical monitoring.

43. OSHA's Hazardous Communication Standard is concerned with preventing occupational exposure to dangerous
    A. diseases.
    B. chemicals.
    C. patients.
    D. procedures.

Infection Control

44. Which of the following conditions could cause poor healing after oral surgery?
    A. Well-controlled diabetes
    B. Poorly controlled diabetes
    C. Dental caries
    D. Arthritis

45. The best way to ensure immunity is by
    A. vaccination.
    B. getting sick.
    C. developing antibodies.
    D. developing allergens.

46. Which of the following diseases is easily transmitted in the healthcare setting?
    A. HIV/AIDS
    B. Tuberculosis
    C. MRSA
    D. Hepatitis A

47. What is the mechanism of action of the autoclave sterilizer?
    A. Dry heat
    B. Steam under pressure
    C. Chemical vapor under pressure
    D. Chemical action

48. The first handwashing of each day should include a
    A. hot water rinse.
    B. soft brush to scrub nails.
    C. quick cold water rinse.
    D. 10-minute surgical prep.

49. Extracted teeth are
    A. medical waste.
    B. regulated waste.
    C. nonregulated waste.
    D. general waste.

50. According to OSHA, the Hepatitis B vaccine is to be made available to employees at risk for contamination. The employee is responsible for
    A. the cost of the vaccine only.
    B. the cost of the vaccine and the office visit.
    C. arriving on time for the appointment.
    D. taking an immune globulin drug.

51. Which of the following procedures is relevant to OSHA's Bloodborne Pathogen Standard?
    A. Secondary labeling
    B. Eyewash stations
    C. Hepatitis B immunization
    D. Patient confidentiality

52. Approximately how much of the waste generated in the dental office is hazardous?
    A. 3%
    B. 10%
    C. 25%
    D. 40%

53. The main disadvantage of using a dry heat sterilizer is the
    A. damage to heat-sensitive items.
    B. corroding of carbon steel instruments.
    C. inability to use closed containers.
    D. inability to use spore testing.

54. Gauze that has had contact with bodily fluids, such as blood and/or saliva, is what type of waste?
    A. Contaminated
    B. Medical
    C. Infectious
    D. Pathogenic

55. Which of the following PPE (personal protective equipment) is used to prevent inhalation of droplets and/or spatter?
    A. Overgloves
    B. Protective eyewear
    C. Mask
    D. Face shield

56. What is the purpose of a barrier in infection control?
    A. Provide an exit portal for infectious agents
    B. Disrupt the transfer of infectious agents
    C. Provide a reservoir for infectious agents
    D. Sterilize infectious agents

57. Used barriers and paper from the dental office are classified as what type of waste?
    A. Regulated
    B. Nonregulated
    C. Biohazardous
    D. Pathogenic

58. Bacteria that must have oxygen to grow and live are considered
    A. anaerobic bacteria.
    B. aerobic bacteria.
    C. facultative bacteria.
    D. gram-positive bacteria.

59. When bacteria form a protective coat of protein around themselves, they are known as
    A. fungi.
    B. viruses.
    C. spores.
    D. protozoa.

60. Which of the following may be used as a surface disinfectant in the dental office?
    A. Iodophors
    B. Ethyl alcohol
    C. Isopropyl alcohol
    D. Ammonia

61. Routine handwashing will remove
    A. resident microflora.
    B. transient microflora.
    C. microbial microflora.
    D. resistant microflora

62. Which of the following is a pathogenic waste?
    A. Mixed amalgam
    B. Needles
    C. Extracted teeth
    D. Spore test strips

63. Any reusable item intended for patient care should be
    A. covered to prevent contamination.
    B. lubricated prior to the next use.
    C. wiped thoroughly with a surface disinfectant.
    D. heat sterilized after use.

64. Of the following choices, which one would reflect the purpose of OSHA Standards MOST accurately?
    A. It is the law and enforceable.
    B. It depends on the state.
    C. It only applies to healthcare.
    D. It is a strong recommendation.

65. The primary advantage of using disposable items in a dental office is
    A. low cost.
    B. reduced cross-contamination.
    C. biodegradability.
    D. bulk quantities.

66. Which of the following chemicals can be used as an immersion disinfectant/sterilant for instruments?
    A. Iodophor
    B. Glutaraldehyde
    C. Sodium hypochlorite
    D. Synthetic phenols

67. What is the appropriate PPE when processing instruments in the ultrasonic cleaner?
    A. Examination gloves, mask, safety glasses, and gown
    B. Overgloves, mask, safety glasses, and gown
    C. Utility gloves, mask, safety glasses, and gown
    D. Double examination gloves, mask, safety glasses, and gown

68. An infection with a short duration is called
    A. chronic.
    B. latent.
    C. acute.
    D. opportunistic.

69. A needlestick injury could transmit disease. This type of disease transmission is called
    A. enteral.
    B. parenteral.
    C. opportunistic.
    D. vector-borne.

70. After treatment, using a low-level disinfectant-type cleaner on the bagged dental chair
    A. is not necessary.
    B. results in microbial resistance.
    C. provides additional asepsis.
    D. requires a second disinfecting.

71. Which of the following actions is MOST appropriate during an OSHA inspection?
    A. Refusal to allow inspector in the office until an attorney is contacted
    B. Offering as much information as possible
    C. Compliance with inspector, without volunteering information
    D. Shadowing the inspector

72. Which of the following is the best choice for cleaning the dental vacuum system?
    A. Nonfoaming, enzymatic cleaner
    B. Bleach solution
    C. Water-based detergent
    D. Chlorhexidine solution

73. Prior to placing instruments into a sterilizer, they must be precleaned in a/an
    A. disinfectant.
    B. autoclave.
    C. ultrasonic unit.
    D. holding solution.

74. Which of the following organizations is the authority for infection control education?
    A. Environment Protection Agency
    B. American Dental Association
    C. Organization for Safety and Asepsis Procedures
    D. Centers for Disease Control and Prevention

75. Which of the following is the MOST effective mouth rinse to use prior to a dental appointment?
    A. Salt water
    B. Chlorhexidine
    C. Mouthwash
    D. Water

76. Which of the following is the LEAST likely route to a hazardous chemical exposure?
    A. Inhalation
    B. Mucous membrane splash
    C. Ingestion
    D. Direct contact

77. Which of the following surface disinfectants is tuberculocidal?
    A. Iodophor
    B. Glutaraldehyde
    C. Bleach
    D. Quaternary ammonia

78. Which surface is likely to become contaminated in a dental operatory during a procedure?
    A. Floor around the chair
    B. Clinical contact surfaces
    C. Patient records
    D. Radiographic equipment

79. Which of the following is a noncritical instrument?
    A. Amalgam condenser
    B. Scalpel
    C. Mouth mirror
    D. X-ray tubehead

80. An example of a percutaneous injury is
   A. aerosol spatter from the high-speed handpiece.
   B. a needlestick from a sharps container.
   C. direct contact with an open lesion.
   D. splatter of a chemical into the eye.

81. If mercury is spilled in the office, it should be cleaned up using a/an
   A. vacuum cleaner.
   B. high-volume evacuator.
   C. spill kit.
   D. x-ray fixer.

82. Which of the following items produces the most aerosol and splatter?
   A. Saliva ejector
   B. High-speed handpiece
   C. Air-water syringe
   D. High-volume evacuator

83. Scrap amalgam should be
   A. disposed of in the trash.
   B. stored in an airtight container.
   C. autoclaved prior to recycling.
   D. burned in an incinerator.

84. *Legionella* bacteria can cause what type of infection in humans?
   A. Cirrhosis
   B. Dermatitis
   C. Intestinal
   D. Pneumonia

85. The purpose of the ultrasonic cleaner is to
   A. disinfect instruments prior to sterilization.
   B. remove debris from instruments prior to sterilization.
   C. sterilize heat-sensitive instruments.
   D. prevent instruments from corrosion.

86. Instruments used on amalgam restorations should be cleaned of all debris prior to autoclaving because amalgam
   A. releases free vapor when heated.
   B. will bake onto the instrument when heated.
   C. can cause cross-contamination.
   D. can harbor microbes.

87. The last PPE put on before beginning patient treatment must be the
   A. mask.
   B. face shield.
   C. gloves.
   D. protective eyewear.
   E. disposable gown.

88. Nitrous oxide exposure in the dental office can be reduced by
   A. using a rubber dam with nitrous patients.
   B. using a ventilation fan in the office.
   C. using a scavenger system.
   D. allowing the patient to talk during treatment.

89. Who is MOST likely to be a susceptible host to pathogenic agents?
    A. Child
    B. Pregnant woman
    C. Person with HIV
    D. Senior citizen

90. The main goal of an effective infection control plan in a dental office is to
    A. reduce the number of microbes.
    B. identify patients with diseases.
    C. assure patients that the office is clean.
    D. keep employees healthy.

91. Items that cannot be placed in the autoclave but are reusable are classified as
    A. critical items.
    B. semicritical items.
    C. noncritical items.
    D. housekeeping items.

92. Orthodontic bands and wires, burs, scalpel blades, and suture needles are
    A. sharps.
    B. disposables.
    C. autoclavable.
    D. reusable.

93. Potable water is another name for
    A. sterilized water.
    B. drinking water.
    C. distilled water.
    D. noningestible water.

94. Which of the following is a required safety measure when using a curing light?
    A. Face mask
    B. Clear safety glasses
    C. Tinted safety glasses
    D. Full face shield

95. To be effective, surface barriers should be
    A. reusable.
    B. fluid resistant.
    C. EPA approved.
    D. sporicidal.

96. Patients who close their lips around the saliva ejector to clear their mouths run the risk of what type of contamination?
    A. Staff to patient
    B. Patient to staff
    C. Patient to patient
    D. Office to community

97. The MOST resistant form of known life is a/an
    A. virulent fungus.
    B. capsule.
    C. spore.
    D. anaerobe.

Infection Control

98. How would a dental assistant ensure that cross-contamination does not occur when a patient's denture is polished in the lab?
    A. Soak the denture in a mouth rinse for 30 minutes.
    B. Have the patient rinse with chlorhexidine for 30 seconds before removing denture.
    C. Use only disposable or sterilized polishing materials.
    D. Disinfect using the spray-wipe-spray technique.

99. How often should a face mask be replaced?
    A. Between patients
    B. Every 30 minutes
    C. Upon completion of each procedure
    D. Once a day

100. The name of the cleaning technique used at the end of a patient appointment is the
    A. spray-wipe-spray.
    B. spray-spray-wipe.
    C. clean-wipe-disinfect.
    D. disinfect-wipe-bag.

See p. 142 for the correct answers and rationales.

Infection Control

ANSWERS AND RATIONALES:
General Chairside (GC)

1. A vasoconstrictor is added to a local anesthetic because it

   C. lengthens the duration of action of the local anesthetic. A vasoconstrictor works by constricting the blood vessels, therefore causing the anesthetic to take longer to travel through the vessels.

2. Which of the following may increase the risk of prolonged bleeding for patients?

   C. Aspirin. Aspirin has the side effect of causing the blood to thin, therefore causing an increase in clotting time.

3. Which cement is exothermic and must be mixed on a glass slab?

   D. Zinc phosphate. When zinc phosphate cement is mixed, a chemical reaction occurs and heat is released. Mixing the cement on a glass slab allows the heat to dissipate, which slows the setting time of the cement.

4. Glass ionomer cement differs from other cements in the unique property of

   B. releasing fluoride. Glass ionomer cement has the ability to release fluoride ions, which prevents secondary decay.

5. After receiving a gel or foam fluoride treatment, how long should a patient wait before eating or drinking?

   C. 30 minutes. Fluoride gels and foams are easily rinsed away from the tooth surface, so waiting 30 minutes before eating or drinking increases their effectiveness.

6. When assembled and positioned properly, the smaller circumference of the matrix band should face which surface of the tooth?

   B. Cervical. A tooth is narrower at the cervix than it is at the occlusal; therefore, the smaller circumference of the matrix band is placed along the gingiva.

7. Who has legal ownership of all patient records and radiographs?

   A. Dentist. Although patients have the right to access and request copies of their personal records and radiographs, the dentist has legal ownership of all records and radiographs.

8. Following the removal of orthodontic brackets, which handpiece is used to remove the bonding material from the tooth?

   B. Ultrasonic. An ultrasonic handpiece is used to remove calculus and stain or to remove bonding materials after orthodontic appliances are removed.

9. An indicator that the final setting time of dental stone has been reached is that the model will be

   D. cool and dry. After an impression is poured, the stone material will start to harden while it goes through an exothermic reaction. During this time, the model will feel warm and damp to the touch. When the model has reached its final set, it will be cool and dry, and the impression can then be removed from the model.

10. A patient suffering from hypoglycemia may exhibit which symptom?

    D. Perspiration. A patient suffering from hypoglycemia may experience perspiration, confusion, increased anxiety, and mood changes.

11. The purpose of inverting the dental dam is to

    D. prevent salivary leakage. Inverting the dental dam creates a seal that will aid in the prevention of salivary leakage.

12. Upon completion of an amalgam restoration, excess amalgam should be disposed of in

    C. a closed container. Excess amalgam has the potential to release mercury vapors into the air. Therefore, it should be stored in a closed container and disposed of according to local and state regulations.

13. An advantage of a diamond bur compared to other dental burs is its

    B. superior cutting edge. Diamond burs have a very hard cutting edge that can be used to cut carious material, tooth material and bone restorations, and appliances. Over time, the diamonds in the grit begin to dislodge, and the grit loses its effectiveness.

14. A deficiency in which of the following vitamins may contribute to night blindness?

    A. Vitamin A. Vitamin A, also known as retinol, is essential for the formation of epithelium, skin, and mucous membranes. It is also necessary to maintain healthy eyes.

15. Which of the following teeth has two roots?

    C. Maxillary first premolar. The maxillary first premolars are the only premolars in the mouth that have two roots. All of the other premolars have only one root.

16. The purpose of attaching a ligature to a dental dam clamp is to

    B. retrieve the clamp if it becomes dislodged and swallowed. A ligature is attached to a dental dam clamp for safety purposes. The ligature will allow the operator or assistant the ability to retrieve a clamp if it becomes dislodged and swallowed or aspirated.

17. Patients requiring oral prophylactic antibiotics prior to a procedure should administer the recommended dose at what time?

    B. 30–60 minutes prior to the procedure. If patients take an oral prophylactic antibiotic 30-60 minutes prior to the dental appointment, it will allow enough time for the antibiotic to enter the bloodstream.

18. The injection technique most preferred by dentists on the mandibular arch is

B. inferior alveolar nerve block. Due to the nature of the mandibular bone being dense and compact, anesthesia is most often delivered using a nerve block injection technique.

19. Which of the following gypsum products has the highest water-to-powder ratio and is the weakest product?

B. Type II: model plaster. Forty-five to 50 ml of water is used when mixing 100 g of model plaster in order to achieve the correct consistency. Model plaster requires the highest water-to-powder ratio.

20. Aspiration allows the dentist to determine the

A. correct placement of the anesthetic. Prior to delivering the local anesthetic into the injection site, the dentist will aspirate to determine whether or not the anesthetic is being injected into a vessel. If during aspiration a small amount of blood is seen in the cartridge, the dentist will reposition the needle before giving the injection.

21. Which of the following is the proper way to make a correction on a patient's chart?

C. Place a single line through the incorrect information and enter the new information on the next line. A patient's chart is a legal document. Never use white-out or erase the information.

22. Which type of anesthesia is frequently used on mandibular teeth and injected near a major nerve in order to numb the entire area served by that nerve branch?

A. Block. Block anesthesia is injected near the nerve trunk of larger terminal nerve branches. It is appropriate for procedures involving teeth or bone on the maxillary and mandibular anterior areas.

23. Which of the following nutrients plays a major role in the development of caries?

D. Carbohydrates. Carbohydrates are broken down into sugars in the mouth by the enzyme salivary amylase.

24. The purpose of applying a topical anesthetic prior to an injection is to

C. desensitize the area. Topical anesthetics will desensitize the oral mucosa and nerve endings to prevent pain during injection.

25. The examination technique that involves the operator using fingers and hands to evaluate hard and soft tissue is called

B. palpation. Palpation is used to evaluate the head, neck, and oral cavity. When palpation is used, the operator is feeling for texture, size, and consistency of the tissues.

26. What accessory is required to attach an abrasive disc to a handpiece?

D. Mandrel. Abrasive discs are attached to a mandrel and then to the handpiece. A mandrel is a metal shaft that is inserted into a low- or high-speed handpiece.

27. Which of the following dental materials can be used as a desensitizer?

    C. Fluoride. Fluoride is used as a desensitizing agent after periodontal treatment and for treatment of dentinal hypersensitivity.

28. Treatment for accidental fluoride overdose includes giving the patient

    C. milk. The calcium in milk acts as a binder for fluoride and will also dilute the fluoride compound in the stomach.

29. When dry, a properly etched enamel surface will appear

    B. chalky. Properly etched enamel will appear chalky white. If the enamel doesn't appear chalky white, the area must be re-etched.

30. What is the primary advantage of adding base metals to noble metals in gold-noble alloys?

    B. Increased resistance to wear. Noble metals are resistant to tarnish and corrosion, and base metals are hard and resistant to wear, so the addition of base metals to noble metals increases wear resistance in gold-noble alloys.

31. Class II restorations are found on

    B. posterior teeth. Class II restorations are found on the molars and premolars, or the posterior teeth.

32. Which method of toothbrushing emphasizes placing the bristles at a 45-degree angle to the sulcus?

    D. Bass. The Bass technique is effective at removing plaque from the gingival margin and is easy for patients to learn.

33. Decay located in the pits and fissures of the occlusal surfaces of molars and premolars are considered which classification of caries?

    A. Class I. Class I caries include pit and fissure cavities in occlusal surfaces of posterior teeth (premolars and molars), buccal and lingual pits on molars, and lingual pits near the cingulum of the maxillary incisors.

34. The material of choice for Class III and Class IV restorations is

    A. composite resin. Composite resin is used for Class III and Class IV restorations on the anterior teeth for esthetic purposes.

35. Which of the following is the most appropriate indication for the application of dental sealants?

    C. Posterior teeth with pits and fissures. Posterior teeth have deep pits and fissures on the occlusal surface, making these areas more susceptible to caries formation because they are difficult to clean.

36. Protective bases can be used to prevent

    C. postoperative sensitivity and damage to the pulp. Protective bases are placed when it is necessary to protect the pulp before the restoration is placed, because without this protection, there may be postoperative sensitivity and damage to the pulp.

37. The purpose of retention pins in restorations is to

B. support core build-ups. A retention pin is anchored into the dentin of the tooth and placed underneath the core build-up.

38. Initial patient contact begins when

B. the patient calls for a new patient appointment. The very first contact a new patient has with the office, whether by phone or in person, will set the tone for the relationship that develops between the office and the patient.

39. The significance of the smear layer in restorative dentistry is to

B. decrease bonding strength. The smear layer is a very thin layer of debris left on the dentin after cavity preparation, which can interfere with bonding agents.

40. Chronic overexposure to low concentrations of fluoride in children younger than 6 years of age will most likely cause which of the following conditions?

D. Dental fluorosis. Dental fluorosis will most likely occur when children experience chronic over-exposure to fluoride, even at low concentrations. Acute fluoride poisoning, although rare, occurs when a high concentration of fluoride gel or solution is accidentally ingested. Anaphylaxis is an allergic reaction occurring immediately following an exposure or injection of an allergen. Decalcification is the beginning of tooth decay occurring on the outside surface of the tooth.

41. A good way to keep the mouth mirror from fogging while the operator is working is to

A. blow some air on it. A light stream of air on the mouth mirror will reduce fogging and remove water or debris that might fall on the mirror and impede the operator's vision.

42. Using the Universal Numbering System, the maxillary right second premolar is designated tooth number

A. 4. The maxillary right second premolar is considered tooth 4. Tooth 5 is the maxillary right first premolar, tooth 12 is the maxillary left first premolar, and tooth 13 is the maxillary left second premolar.

43. Treatment of alveolitis includes

C. irrigation with a saline solution. Alveolitis or dry socket is irrigated with warm saline solution, and a strip of iodoform gauze is packed into the socket to help prevent infection and promote healing.

44. Calcium hydroxide can be used for all of the following purposes EXCEPT as a

D. dental varnish. Calcium hydroxide can be used as a temporary cement, base, or restorative material based on the thickness of the mix. Copal resin or fluorides are used as varnishes.

45. When assisting a right-handed dentist, the dental assistant would use the right hand for

D. operating the high-volume evacuator. While using the one-handed exchange of instrument transfer, the left hand is making the instrument transfers while the right hand is holding the high-volume evacuator, retracting tissues, or preparing the next instruments or materials needed.

46. A rapid change in body position, such as when the patient is suddenly placed in the upright position, may result in

   B. postural hypotension. Postural hypotension, also called orthostatic hypotension, occurs when there is an insufficient amount of blood flow to the brain. This condition can occur in a patient immediately after a sudden change in positioning, such as after being reclined in the dental chair for a period of time and then brought to an upright position too fast.

47. When placing the Tofflemire retainer around a tooth, the diagonal slot should face toward the

   A. gingival surface. The diagonal slot of the Tofflemire retainer should always be positioned facing the gingiva. This enables the operator to slide the retainer off the tooth after the restoration has been placed, allowing the band to remain in place without harming the patient's tissues.

48. What can be used as a visual aid to show the patient the areas in the mouth where debris remains after brushing and flossing?

   B. Disclosing agent. A disclosing agent identifies bacterial plaque deposits on the teeth and oral tissues, which might otherwise be invisible. After staining, the plaque deposits can be seen distinctly and aid in patient instruction.

49. To prevent the patient from accidentally swallowing the rubber dam clamp, affix

   D. a piece of dental floss around the clamp. Tie a piece of dental floss to the bow of the clamp so the clamp can be retrieved if it becomes dislodged. Also, the floss can be anchored onto the dental dam frame once the complete dam setup is in place in the oral cavity for extra precaution while working.

50. On a prescription, the abbreviation q.i.d. means

   D. four times a day. The abbreviation q.i.d stands for *quater in die* in Latin and means four times a day.

51. Which of the following instruments is used to remove caries during a restorative procedure?

   B. Round cutting bur. Round cutting burs are used to remove caries. Gingival margin trimmers and enamel hatchets are used in the preparation of the cavity floor and walls after the removal of the dental decay (caries). Curettes are periodontal instruments, not restorative instruments.

52. Which of the following materials would be placed into the prepared tooth FIRST for an amalgam restoration?

   D. Calcium hydroxide. Using the materials listed, the first material placed into the prepared tooth is the liner (calcium hydroxide) followed by the cavity varnish (copal resin). The base material (glass ionomer cement) is placed after the varnish and the amalgam is last.

53. If the dentist is running behind schedule, patients that are waiting for their appointment should be

   C. informed of the situation. Whenever the office is running behind schedule, the patient should be informed and the patient can then decide to wait or reschedule the appointment.

54. The cementum, alveolar bone, and gingiva are part of the

   D. periodontium. The periodontium refers to the tissues that surround and support the tooth.

55. Antihistamines are used for treating

    C. allergic reactions. Antihistamines include drugs that counteract the effects of histamine, which plays a key role in causing an allergic reaction. Examples of antihistamines commonly used are Benadryl, Dramamine, Claritin, and Chlor-Trimeton.

56. Bitewing radiographs show that there is decay under an existing restoration. This type of caries is called

    B. recurrent caries. Recurrent caries occur under or near the margins of an existing tooth restoration.

57. Varnishes are commonly used in amalgam cavity preparations to

    A. seal and protect the dentin from migration of agents into the tooth. Varnish is most commonly used as a sealer of the dentinal tubules in an amalgam preparation. This helps prevent the outward migration of other restorative materials—that is, acidic liner, cement base, or metallic ions—from the amalgam from damaging the tooth.

58. When teaching toothbrushing, the emphasis should be on brushing

    D. until complete removal of plaque regardless of time. The main consideration in effective tooth brushing is the thorough removal of bacterial plaque and other soft debris from the tooth surfaces and oral tissues rather than the number of brushings. How frequent, as well as the number of tooth brushing strokes or amount of time spent accomplishing the task, ultimately depends on the patient's ability and efficiency.

59. During an amalgam restoration procedure, articulating paper is used to evaluate the

    C. occlusion after carving. Articulating paper is used to check the occlusion. The patient is instructed to bite gently on the articulating paper. Heavy marks will appear when there are high spots on the new restoration. The dentist will then use a carver or finishing bur to remove the high spots. This step is repeated as necessary until the new restoration is brought into proper occlusion.

60. If all of the normal treatments for angina do not relieve the pain that the patient is experiencing, the dental team should assume that the patient is suffering from

    A. myocardial infarction. If the patient is suffering from angina, nitroglycerin will relieve the symptoms. If nitroglycerin doesn't relieve the pain within a few minutes, the patient may be having a heart attack, and emergency services should be called.

61. What is used during a crown and bridge preparation to displace the gingival tissue?

    B. Retraction cord. Gingival retraction cord is used to temporarily displace the gingival tissue and widen the sulcus so that the impression material can flow around all parts of the tooth preparation.

62. Which of the following may be seen in a patient with bulimia?

    C. Erosion of the lingual surfaces of the teeth. A patient with bulimia may show signs of erosion on the lingual surfaces of the teeth, particularly the maxillary anteriors. This is due to the acid produced by frequent vomiting.

63. After spraying an impression with disinfectant, the impression should be

    B. sealed in a plastic bag. After thoroughly spraying an impression with disinfectant, it should be wrapped in a well-moistened paper towel and stored in a covered container or sealed in a plastic bag until pouring can be accomplished.

64. Antibiotic premedication is recommended for patients who may be susceptible for

    B. developing infective endocarditis. Patients who are prescribed antibiotic premedication are those who have a medical condition that can make them highly susceptible for developing infective endocarditis, such as rheumatic heart disease and congenital heart defects.

65. Which of the following conditions may occur if excess cement is not removed from the cervical margin after cementation of a crown?

    C. Inflammation of interdental papilla. Excess cement that remains around the margins of a crown will act as a chronic mechanical irritant to the gingival tissues, resulting in gingival inflammation.

66. The surgical instrument used to trim alveolar bone and eliminate sharp bony projections is a

    C. rongeur. The rongeur is similar in size to extraction forceps and resembles nail clippers with sharp cutting edges, but it also has a spring between the handles.

67. Xerostomia refers to

    A. dryness of the mouth. Xerostomia is caused by the absence or diminished amount of saliva. Xerostomia is a contributing factor in oral discomfort and dental caries.

68. A veneer is applied to which surface of a prepared tooth?

    B. Facial. Veneers are placed on the outer surface of the tooth to improve its appearance, such as treating darkened or yellowed teeth, as well as to repair tooth abnormalities, such as crooked or misshapen teeth.

69. The primary dentition contains how many premolars?

    A. 0. Unlike the permanent dentition, which contains 4 premolars in each arch, the primary dentition does not contain any premolars. Upon exfoliation, the primary molars are replaced by the permanent premolars.

70. When placing dental cement for a crown or veneer, the assistant should coat the

    C. restoration with a thin layer of material. An indirect restoration requires a cement mixed to a luting consistency. If the material is too thick, the restoration will not seat properly. Ideally, the luting material should be thin enough to flow when a thin layer coats the interior of the restoration for seating.

71. Which of the following instruments is used to carve the interproximal portion of an amalgam restoration?

    D. Hollenback. The Hollenback carver is an interproximal carver used to contour or remove excess amalgam from the proximal surfaces of the restoration.

72. Which of the following is part of a full maxillary denture?

    B. Post dam. Retention of a maxillary denture relies on a suction seal to keep it in place. This is known as the post dam.

73. What is the treatment for angina pectoris?

    D. Nitroglycerin. Nitroglycerin is the common medication indicated for the immediate relief of heart pain, particularly angina pectoris.

74. What is used to determine the color of the composite resin material during the restorative procedure?

    E. Shade guide. A shade guide is used to match the composite resin material to the color of the natural tooth.

75. Which filler type of composite resin has the strongest makeup and is used commonly for posterior restorations?

    B. Macrofilled. Macrofilled composites, also known as the traditional or conventional composite materials, are composed of the largest filler particles and are the strongest of the composite resins. Because of their strength, the macrofilled composites are commonly used for posterior restorations where greater strength and fracture resistance is important

76. The goal of water fluoridation is to adjust the fluoride content to

    C. 1.0 ppm. Water fluoridation is the addition of fluoride ions to achieve optimal fluoridation of approximately 1 ppm.

77. All of the following instruments are required for packing retraction cord EXCEPT for

    C. a discoid cleoid. In addition to a basic setup (mirror, explorer, and cotton pliers), a cord-packing instrument is required for packing gingival retraction cord. The discoid cleoid instrument is a restorative instrument used for carving amalgam.

78. The charting symbol illustrated between tooth number 28 and tooth number 29 designates

    C. open contact. The charting symbol used to designate an open contact is two blue or black short vertical parallel lines drawn between two adjacent teeth.

79. The charting symbol illustrated on tooth number 24 indicates

    D. root canal. A blue or black line drawn through the center of each root of a tooth indicates that the tooth has a root canal.

80. Which of the following conditions exist between tooth number 8 and tooth number 9?

    C. Diastema. A diastema is a large open contact/space that can occur between maxillary central incisors. This condition is usually charted as two black or blue vertical parallel lines drawn between the two teeth where the space exists.

81. Which of the following restorations is charted on tooth number 29?

    B. Stainless steel crown. When charting a tooth that has been restored using a stainless steel crown, the letters "SS" are printed in either blue or black on the occlusal surface of the tooth.

82. Which of the following conditions exists on the permanent maxillary left central incisor?

    D. Implant. Horizontal black or blue lines drawn through the root or roots of a tooth indicate an existing implant.

83. Which of the following actions should be taken first in managing an office emergency?

    A. Calling for EMS. Activation of the EMS should always be the first step in management of an emergency.

84. During a composite procedure, sectional matrices are used in conjunction with which of the following?

    B. Tension ring. Sectional matrix systems require the use of a tension ring with the small, oval-shaped stainless steel matrix band.

85. The primary objective of amalgam polishing is to

    C. create a smoother surface with fewer irregularities. Although amalgam polishing helps to improve the cosmetic appearance of amalgam restorations, the primary objective is to remove surface irregularities and create a smoother surface. By doing so, bacterial plaque and food debris are less apt to adhere to the restoration.

86. An accurate record of a patient's financial history with the dental office should be recorded

    B. on a manual or electronic ledger card. All patient financial transactions, including treatment charges and payments, should be recorded on the patient's ledger card in order to keep accurate records.

87. Topical anesthetic is applied prior to giving an injection in order to

    D. desensitize the tissue at the injection site. The primary purpose of a topical anesthetic is to provide a temporary numbing effect at the injection site before the local anesthetic is administered.

88. In an emergency, check the patient for a pulse at which artery?

    D. Carotid. The American Red Cross and The American Heart Association recommend that rescuers check the carotid artery in the patient's neck for a pulse.

89. If a right-handed operator is preparing tooth number 3 for a crown, the dental assistant would place the bevel of the high-velocity evacuator

    B. parallel to the lingual surface of the tooth being prepared. Preparing tooth number 3 would require the dental assistant to place the bevel of the high-velocity evacuator parallel to the lingual surface while retracting the patient's cheek.

90. The primary cause of syncope (fainting) in the dental office is

   A. allergic reaction to local anesthetic. Pain, fear, disease, and other factors will increase a patient's anxiety level. Anxiety is the primary cause of a patient losing consciousness while in the dental office.

91. During an amalgam procedure, which instrument is used to pack the amalgam firmly into the tooth preparation?

   B. Condenser. Amalgam condensers use manual pressure to tightly "condense" the amalgam into the tooth preparation, increasing the strength of the restoration.

92. Which of the following is associated with the intake of sugar-free sodas and dental caries?

   D. An increase in acidity. Although diet sodas may be sugar free, they contain phosphoric acid, resulting in a pH value lower than 3.5 and highly acidic. The critical pH for enamel demineralization and the development of dental caries averages 4.5 to 5.5. The amount of demineralization and extent of dental caries also depends on the length of time and the frequency with which an acid with a pH below the critical pH is in contact with tooth surfaces.

93. The properly seated dental assistant is

   C. 4 to 6 in above the dentist. The dental assistant should sit 4 to 6 in above the operator in order to see over his or her hands and into the patient's mouth.

94. Calcium hydroxide is used under new restorations to

   D. stimulate reparative dentin. When the preparation is deep, calcium hydroxide stimulates the odontoblasts that lie between the pulp and dentin to facilitate the formation of reparative dentin.

95. Subgingival calculus is removed using a

   A. curette. The curette differs from other scalers in that it has a rounded tip to allow the instrument to work under the gingiva to remove calculus and smooth rough surfaces.

96. Impressions should be disinfected

   B. at the chairside upon removal. Ideally, disinfection of impressions should begin in the operatory through chairside measures once the impression is removed from the mouth.

97. Which of the following choices represents the lowest ratio, meaning greatest concentration, of vasoconstrictor in local anesthetic?

   A. 1:20,000. The greatest concentration of vasoconstrictor found in a local anesthetic is 1:20,000. A smaller ratio indicates a higher percentage of vasoconstrictor. In most situations, it is desirable to use the *highest* ratio (lowest concentration of vasoconstrictor) possible.

98. The attachments at the sides of a three-unit bridge are called

   B. abutments. An abutment is used to support and retain a fixed or removable prosthesis.

99. Which of the following refers to an allergic response that could threaten a patient's life?

   C. Anaphylaxis. A life-threatening allergic response is known as anaphylaxis. This may cause the tongue to swell and block the airway preventing the patient from breathing.

100. A patient with dental insurance is classified as the

   C. subscriber. When a person has dental insurance that pays for a portion of his or her dental treatment, he or she is known as the subscriber.

101. The portion of the bridge that replaces the missing tooth is the

   A. pontic. A pontic is an artificial tooth that replaces a missing tooth.

102. To minimize a patient's gag reflex while taking a maxillary alginate impression, the dental assistant would use

   B. hot water and fast-set material. Fast-set alginate requires a faster mixing time and will set up in the patient's mouth at a faster rate. Warm water allows impression material to set up faster as well.

103. The operator has prepared an MO amalgam preparation on tooth number 3. The interproximal box is rough and needs to be smoothed. What would you pass to the operator?

   D. Enamel hatchet. Hatchets are used to cut and smooth the walls and floors of the preparation.

104. When should sealants be placed on a tooth?

   B. As soon as the tooth has fully erupted. Pit and fissure sealants should be placed on newly erupted teeth and those free of decay. The highest risk for decay is generally within the first 3 years of eruption.

105. During an operative procedure, the best way to keep the tooth from overheating and damaging the pulp is to

   B. spray a mixture of air and water over the tooth. A water spray will help cool the tooth and remove debris as the operator prepares the tooth for the restoration.

106. A patient who begins to breathe deeply and rapidly is experiencing

   B. hyperventilation. Hyperventilation, or over breathing, is the result of a stressful situation. Individuals will experience numbness around the mouth, light headedness, and dizziness from a lack of CO_2 in the system.

107. Which wall of the cavity preparation is perpendicular to the long axis of the tooth?

   D. Pulpal wall. The pulpal wall, also known as the pulpal floor, is a horizontal wall of the preparation that intersects with the line of the long axis of the tooth.

108. Which classification of restoration does NOT require a matrix band?

   A. I. The Class I restoration does not require a matrix band because there is no interproximal area to restore.

109. When punching a rubber dam for a restorative procedure, the anchor tooth should be

    C. 1 or 2 teeth to the distal. The rubber dam clamp should be placed 1 or 2 teeth distal to the tooth to be prepared so the anchor hole is punched to match the clamped tooth.

110. During an emergency, the AED is used to provide which of the following to the heart?

    C. Electricity. The AED (automated external defibrillator) is an advanced microprocessor used to monitor the patient's heart rhythm and automatically defibrillate if necessary. In defibrillation, an electrical shock is sent to the heart muscle to help reestablish the proper rhythm of the heart.

111. The agents that provide a temporary numbing effect on nerve endings located on the surface of the oral mucosa are

    B. topical anesthetics. Topical anesthetics provide a temporary numbing effect on nerve endings located on the surface of the oral mucosa, such as where an injection is to take place.

112. Mrs. Applebee recently had an MOD amalgam placed in tooth number 14. Her tooth was temperature sensitive for about a week and then the sensitivity subsided. This temporary hypersensitivity was most likely due to which of the following?

    B. Pulpal hyperemia. Patients sometimes experience hypersensitivity for a brief period of time after the placement of a direct or indirect restoration. This is most likely due to pulpal hyperemia.

113. What is achieved by injecting the anesthetic solution directly into the tissue at the site of the dental procedure?

    C. Infiltration anesthesia. Infiltration anesthesia is injected near the apex of the tooth, near larger terminal nerve branches, to prevent impulses from passing from the tooth to the central nervous system.

114. Anaphylaxis is considered to be

    B. a life-threatening allergic reaction. Anaphylaxis is considered to be a life-threatening allergic reaction. Emergency care should be administered immediately.

115. During the finishing of a Class III composite restoration, which of the following instruments may be used to remove excess flash and to smooth the interproximal area?

    A. Abrasive strip. A number 12 scalpel blade in an appropriate scalpel blade handle may also be used to help remove the excess flash from the edges of the restoration. Mounted polishing discs, sand paper discs, as well as egg-shaped finishing burs are not suitable for removing flash material from interproximal areas.

116. Hardness of a material is ranked using the

    C. Mohs scale. The Mohs scale ranks materials by their relative resistance to abrasion.

117. Which of the following instruments are NOT used in refining and finishing the cavity walls and margins of the cavity preparation?

    D. Spoon excavators. Spoon excavators and round burs in a low-speed handpiece are used during the process of removing decay from the tooth, not in the preparation/refinement of the prepared tooth.

118. When a patient fails to show for an appointment, the scheduling assistant should

   A. call the patient and summarize the conversation in the patient's chart. Every effort should be made to personally speak to a patient who has missed an appointment. A brief summary is entered into the patient record for future reference.

119. In four-handed dentistry, the area of exchange is located

   A. across the chest near the patient's chin. The transfer zone is the invisible area where the actual exchange of instruments takes place—it's typically below the patient's chin and over their chest.

120. The dental team member most likely to be in charge of calling the emergency medical services is the

   A. business assistant. Most often, it is the business assistant who is assigned the role to call the emergency services during an emergency situation. The business assistant should remain on the telephone until the necessary emergency medical services are obtained.

ANSWERS AND RATIONALES:
Radiation Health and Safety (RHS)

1. Which of the following film speeds is the fastest?

   D. F. F-speed film is 20% faster than E, and E is 50% faster than D. A is the slowest.

2. The purpose of the aluminum filter is to

   C. allow for a more penetrating primary beam. The aluminum filter removes the low-energy, long wavelengths from the primary beam, which produces better penetrating power.

3. Overexposure to a safelight will produce a film that is

   B. fogged. If film is exposed to the safelight for more than 2 to 3 minutes, the film will appear fogged.

4. What describes a radiograph's darkness?

   A. Density. Density describes the opacity of an object to X-rays, with denser objects more opaque.

5. The maximum permissible dose of radiation for an operator is

   D. 5 REMs or 0.05 Sv per year. The National Council on Radiation Protection and Measurements has determined that the maximum permissible dose for an occupationally exposed worker is 5 REMs or 0.05 Sv per year.

6. Areas that appear dark on a radiograph are called

   B. radiolucent. Dark areas on a radiograph are radiolucent. The darker or more radiolucent the structure is, the less dense the structure.

7. Cells with a high reproductive rate are considered to be

   B. radiosensitive. Cells with a high reproductive rate are constantly dividing and reproducing. They are more sensitive to the effects of radiation.

8. A radiograph that is exposed using a high kVp will have

   A. many shades of gray. Using a higher kVp will produce a radiograph with many shades of gray. This type of radiograph has a low contrast.

9. Which of the four components of a film packet reduces secondary radiation?

   D. Lead foil. Radiation is most effectively stopped by lead.

10. The largest intraoral film size is

   D. #4. Intraoral film size #4 is used mostly when exposing an occlusal radiograph on an adult.

11. Which of the following helps reduce the X-ray exposure of a patient?

   C. Collimator. A collimator is a piece of lead that restricts the beam to the size of the film.

12. In radiograph 1, the film was positioned too far

   D. occlusally. When the film was placed in the mouth, it was not positioned far enough up (too far occlusally) to include the roots of the teeth.

13. The technical error in radiograph 2 is an example of

   A. elongation. Both overlapping and elongation can be seen on the premolar and molars in this radiograph.

14. Which technical errors are illustrated in radiographs 3 and 4?

   C. Film placement. The technical error seen in both radiographs 3 and 4 is incorrect film placement. Bitewing films must be positioned so that the resulting radiographic exposures show equal portions of both the maxillary and mandibular crowns of the posterior teeth. The premolar bitewing film needs to be positioned so that the resulting image shows both the maxillary and mandibular premolars, as well as the distal contact areas of the canines. The film must also be positioned so that the front edge of the film includes at least half of the mandibular canine in the resulting image. The molar bitewing film must be positioned so that both the maxillary and mandibular molars are visible on the resulting image. The film also needs to be centered over the mandibular second molar and the front edge of the film must be positioned to include the distal half of the mandibular second premolar in the resulting image.

15. Which of the following is the major advantage of a panoramic radiograph?

   A. Lower cost to the patient compared to intraoral films. A panoramic radiograph includes all teeth in only one film. A complete film series can require 18 to 22 films to capture all of a patient's teeth. The savings of clinician time and film allows a cost savings for the patient.

16. Which of the following structures will appear radiopaque on a radiograph?

   A. PFM. PFM, metal restorations, tooth enamel, and dense areas of bone are examples of radiopaque images.

17. Which of the following anatomical structures will appear radiolucent on a radiograph?

   C. Mental foramen. The mental foramen is an opening in the mandible located near the apical area of the premolars. It will appear radiolucent because it lacks thickness.

18. Which of the following cells are the MOST radiosensitive?

   C. Bone marrow cells. Bone marrow cells have the highest sensitivity to radiation. Muscle and nerve cells have a low sensitivity. Salivary gland cells have a moderately low sensitivity.

19. The number of waves that pass a given point per unit of time is the

   C. wave frequency. Frequency is the measure of the number of waves per unit of time.

20. If a film is reversed in the mouth during an exposure, the resulting image will look

   B. lighter. The resulting image will have a washed out appearance, along with a herringbone or tire tread effect, because the X-ray beam has passed through the piece of lead foil located toward the tab side of the film.

21. The period of time between the exposure to X-rays and the appearance of radiation damage is called the

   B. latent period. The latent period, or the time between radiation exposure and its biologic effects, may be years.

22. Which of the following conditions can be identified on a radiograph?

   C. Salivary stones. Salivary stones and root tips are the only two conditions identifiable on a radiograph because of their density. Herpetic lesions, aphthous ulcers, and frena are composed of soft tissue.

23. Which of the following types of ionizing radiation produce the least amount of scatter radiation?

   B. Short wavelength radiation. Short wavelength radiation is able to penetrate tissue better and produces less scatter radiation.

24. How often should automatic processing solutions be changed?

   C. Every 3 to 4 weeks. Automatic processing solutions should be changed every 3 to 4 weeks. They should be replenished daily.

25. Elongation of an image on a radiograph may be caused by

   A. insufficient vertical angulation. Elongation is caused by insufficient vertical angulation of the tubehead.

26. Regulations state that an X-ray unit operating above 70 kVp must have a total filtration of

   C. 2.5 mm. Any unit that operates at a higher level than 70 kVp must have aluminum filtration of 2.5 mm built into its head.

27. A radiopaque landmark found superimposed over the apical areas of the molars in the maxilla is the

   B. floor of the sinus. The floor of the sinus is located above the maxillary molars and premolars. It appears as a radiopaque structure.

28. When using the bisecting angle technique, the vertical angulation of the maxillary premolar exposure is

   C. +30. All maxillary teeth and structures are exposed using a positive vertical angulation. Angulations can range between approximately 10 degrees difference. Incisors are +40 to +50. Canines are +45 to +55. Premolars are +30 to +40. Molars are +20 to +30.

29. The advantage of using intensifying screens in extraoral radiography is

 A. reduced exposure time. Intensifying screens reduce exposure time, which, in turn, reduces the radiation exposure for the patient during the relatively longer exposure times involved with extraoral radiography.

30. Failure to fix films long enough will result in a radiograph with

 D. a brown tint. A brown tint occurs when the film was not allowed in the fixer bath long enough or the film was not adequately rinsed.

31. The negatively charged part of the X-ray tube is the

 A. cathode. The cathode is the negatively charged end of an X-ray tube where electrons are created by heating a tungsten filament before being shot across the vacuum tube to the anode end.

32. What is the best way for an assistant to evaluate the amount of radiation he or she receives?

 D. Wear a dosimeter at work for 3 months. Dosimeters are worn for 3 months before they are returned to the monitoring company. Film badges monitor radiation, but they should not be worn outside the office.

33. At the patient's skin, the diameter of the X-ray beam should not exceed

 C. 2.75 in. Limiting the diameter of the X-ray beam to 2.75 in reduces the amount of radiation received by the patient.

34. Excessive vertical angulation causes

 A. foreshortened tooth structures. Excessive vertical angulation causes tooth structures to be foreshortened. Elongation is caused by inadequate vertical angulation.

35. Which of the following structures will appear the most radiopaque on a radiograph?

 B. Pulp chamber. Dense structures appear radiopaque (whitish) on a radiograph. Amalgam restorations are metal and quite dense, so they will appear the most radiopaque of all of these structures.

36. If the developer solution is exhausted, the radiograph will be

 B. underdeveloped. A weak or cold developing solution or insufficient developing time will result in an underdeveloped radiograph.

37. Which of the following is a property of X-rays?

 C. They have no mass or weight. X-rays have no mass or weight. Also, they travel at the speed of light, have no charge, and have the ability to cause biological changes in cells.

38. The maximum yearly permissible dose of radiation that a pregnant woman should receive is

 B. 50 mSv (or 5,000 millirem/mrem). A pregnant woman not occupationally exposed to radiation is limited to 10% of that allowed for occupational workers: 50 mSv or 5,000 millirem/mrem.

39. What is the minimum distance an operator should stand during an X-ray exposure?

   B. 6 ft. Ideally, the operator should stand at least 6 ft away, behind the bulkiest part of the patient's head, and between 90 degrees and 135 degrees out of the primary beam.

40. Which of the following would the operator adjust in order to increase the quantity of electrons inside the X-ray tube?

   A. Milliamperage. Milliamperage is a measure of the quantity of electrons generated inside the X-ray tube. The more electrons, the greater the amount of radiation.

41. Overexposure of the skin to radiation will cause a redness or sunburned appearance called

   C. erythema. Erythema is a redness of the skin caused by irritation and/or infection.

42. What must be done with nondisposable dental film holders after each use?

   C. They must be sterilized. Nondisposable dental film holders are semicritical items because they are placed in the patient's mouth and touch mucous membranes. They should be sterilized.

43. The target in the X-ray tube is composed of what metal?

   D. Tungsten. When the exposure button is pressed, a high-voltage circuit is activated that shoots the cloud of electrons across the vacuum tube to a tungsten target on the positive, or anode, side of the X-ray tube.

44. Identify the anatomical structure that will appear radiolucent on a radiograph.

   A. Mental foramen. The mental foramen appears as a radiolucent anatomical structure between the mandibular premolars. The genial tubercles, nasal spine, and external oblique ridge all appear radiopaque.

45. A collar on a lead apron is used to protect the patient's

   B. thyroid gland. A lead collar extends the top of the apron to cover the patient's neck, thereby protecting thyroid tissue that is highly sensitive to radiation.

46. Overlapping images is caused by

   B. incorrect horizontal angulation. Incorrect horizontal angulation results in overlapping images from adjacent teeth, obscuring the interproximal contact areas.

47. What type of X-rays produce the radiographic image in the form of the latent image?

   B. Primary. The interaction of the primary beam of radiation with the film packet produces a latent or hidden image that does not appear until the film is developed.

48. Which of the following is the correct test to detect light leaks in the darkroom?

   B. Coin test. Unwrap a slightly exposed film in the darkroom under safelight conditions. Place a coin on the film for 2 to 3 minutes. Then process the film as normal. If the coin is visible on the film after processing, there is a light leak in the darkroom, leading to film fogging.

Radiation Health and Safety

49. A structure that stops or absorbs X-rays will appear

   B. radiopaque. Radiopaque objects absorb X-ray energy and show up as lighter areas on a radiograph.

50. The most penetrating X-rays have a

   C. short wavelength. The shorter the wavelength, the higher the energy and the greater the penetration power.

51. The RINN XCP is assembled to expose a mandibular right molar periapical. Which of the following areas can be exposed without having to reassemble the film holder?

   B. Maxillary left molar. An XCP assembled to expose a mandibular right molar periapical can also be used to expose a maxillary left molar.

52. On which radiograph would the inverted Y be seen?

   B. Maxillary canine periapical. The inverted Y is a radiopaque structure formed by the outline of the nasal floor and the anterior floor of the maxillary sinus and is seen on the maxillary canine periapical radiograph.

53. ALARA stands for

   C. as low as reasonably achievable. The ALARA principle recommends using the fastest speed film available and as little radiation as is feasible to get a high-quality radiograph.

54. A step-wedge is a device used to test the

   A. automatic processor. Step-wedge devices can be used to check both the automatic process and radiation output.

55. To avoid cone cuts on a radiograph, the operator must

   A. center the PID over the film. A cone cut is the result of the PID not being positioned evenly to the film, resulting in an image that leaves a partial blank space on the exposed film.

56. Assuming that the mA and kVp stay the same, if the focal-film distance doubles, the exposure time needed to produce a quality film quadruples. This concept is known as

   B. inverse square law. The inverse square law is a rule that states the intensity of radiation is inversely proportional to the square of the distance from the source of the radiation. As the distance increases, radiation intensity at the object decreases.

57. When taking a radiographic survey on a child under the age of 10 years, the exposure (mAs) should be reduced by

   C. 50%. Because the pediatric patient is smaller and his or her bone is less dense than the adult patient, the exposure factors (mAs) should be reduced by 50% for children under the age of 10. For children between 10 and 15 years old, the exposure factors (mAs) should be reduced by 25%.

58. Identify the correct setting that would indicate the PID pointing to the floor.

B. +10. Positive angulations indicate the PID is pointing toward the floor. Negative angulations indicate the PID is pointing toward the ceiling.

59. Decreasing the amount of time a duplicating film is exposed to light will result in a film that is

A. darker. The longer the duplicating film is exposed to the light source, the lighter it will be. This is the opposite of X-ray film, which becomes darker with prolonged exposure to X-ray radiation.

60. A size #3 film is used for

B. a bitewing radiograph on an adult. A size #3 film is too big to use on a child and is only made for bitewing exposures.

61. Which of the following is responsible for the recording of the image on the radiograph?

B. Polyester base. When x-radiation strikes the silver halide crystals they are excited and turn black. The more radiation the crystals are exposed to, the blacker they become, producing an image on the film.

62. Which anatomic structure will be present on a mandibular anterior radiograph?

C. Lingual foramen. The lingual foramen will appear on a mandibular anterior radiograph. The mental foramen will appear on a mandibular posterior radiograph. The incisive foramen will appear on a maxillary anterior radiograph. The mandibular foramen is located distal to the third mandibular molar on the internal surface of the mandible.

63. Bitewing radiographs are most useful in diagnosis of

B. interproximal decay. Bitewing films are used to diagnose decay between teeth (e.g., interproximal decay), decay under restorations, faulty restorations, and periodontal bone loss.

64. Bitewing radiographs are used to locate

D. interproximal caries. Bitewing radiographs are used to locate interproximal caries. Periodontal disease, apical lesions, and impacted teeth can be seen on periapical radiographs.

65. Patients are protected from radiation by the filter in the tubehead that

C. eliminates stronger wavelengths. Filtration of X-rays is controlled by aluminum filters in the tubehead, which eliminate the longer, weaker wavelengths that could harm the patient.

66. When processing radiographs manually, the time and temperature for developing is

C. 5 minutes at 68° F. According to manufacturer's instructions, the ideal time and temperature for developing radiographs is 5 minutes at 68° F. Changes to temperature require adjustments in the length of time the films are processed.

67. Film speed is determined by

   C. the size of the crystal. Film speed is determined by the size of the crystals in the emulsion. Milliamperage determines the amount of radiation in the X-ray beam and kilovoltage determines the penetrating power of the X-ray beam. Film size has no bearing on film speed.

68. Radiation that impacts future generations has what kind of effect?

   B. Genetic. Exposure to radiation can have a negative impact on the very sensitive reproductive cells causing genetic defects to occur over time.

69. A correctly placed premolar bitewing will include the

   D. mesial of the canine. The film should be positioned so its leading edge is parallel with the mandibular canine. Incorrect placement will obscure the distal canine surface.

70. The mandibular canal is found on which film?

   D. Mandibular molar PA. The mandibular canal is a radiolucent horizontal canal that is visible below the apex of the mandibular molars as two faint parallel radiopaque lines.

71. In which exposure would one identify the genial tubercle as a landmark?

   C. Mandibular incisor. The genial tubercle is a radiopaque, donut-shaped area that surrounds the lingual foramen.

72. The maxillary tuberosity is found on which film?

   A. Maxillary molar. The maxillary tuberosity is a large area of rounded bone found behind the farthest molar in the maxillary arch.

73. Which of the following anatomical landmarks is not visible in the mandibular molar exposure?

   B. Mental foramen. The mental foramen is visible near the apices of the mandibular first and second premolar and will not be visible in the molar exposure.

74. Compared to ANSI D-speed film, F-speed film

   D. requires less exposure time. F-speed film is the fastest film and, therefore, has less exposure time.

75. Old developing solutions will cause the films to appear

   C. light. After a period of use, developing solutions will become exhausted and need to be changed. Films will appear light and will be very difficult to read.

76. Which of the following can result in a light film?

   C. Reversed film. A reversed film will cause a film to appear light. Exposure to white light will result in a dark film. An unsafe safelight will result in a film that is fogged. Overdevelopment will result in a darker film.

77. The process of removing electrons from atoms is called

   B. ionization. The process of removing electrons from atoms results in ionization. An atom that has gained or lost an electron is known as an ion.

78. This radiograph is an example of which of the following?

   C. Periapical radiograph. Periapical films are used to examine anatomy and pathology in the root area and surrounding bony structures. The image included on the periapical film needs to include the entire length of the teeth of interest, as well 3 to 4 mm of supporting tissue beyond the root apices.

79. What size of film was used for this radiographic exposure?

   C. 2. Size 2 film is typically used for periapical exposures of posterior teeth.

80. The radiopaque areas visible in the mesial and distal roots of the molar are

   D. root canals. Root canals that appear radiopaque are present in the mandibular first molar.

81. The radiopaque material visible in the roots of the mandibular molar is most likely

   B. gutta percha. Gutta percha is a rubber-like substance used to fill a root canal. It comes in the form of cones, called gutta percha points.

82. The restoration visible in the second premolar is a/an

   C. DO amalgam. The restoration on the second molar is a DO amalgam restoration.

83. Which of the following factors determines exposure time?

   C. Size of patient. The position indicating device and the horizontal and vertical angulation do not affect exposure time. The denser the object, the more X-rays needed to penetrate the object, and the more exposure time needed.

84. Correct horizontal angulation prevents which of the following radiographic errors?

   B. Foreshortening. If the horizontal angulation of the PID is correct, then the central beam of the X-ray will be directed through the interdental contacts, preventing overlapping.

85. What is the purpose of a risk management program for taking radiographs in the dental office?

   A. Reduce the chance of a malpractice suit. A risk management program involves policies and procedures that will reduce the chance that a malpractice suit will be brought against the dental office.

86. An X-ray machine operating at 70 kVp must have how much aluminum filtration in order to comply with federal law?

   D. 2.5 mm. Federal requirements for the aluminum filter on an X-ray machine operating at 70 kVp or greater must be 2.5 mm.

87. Static from improperly handling film will appear to have which pattern on the finished film?

   C. Lightening. Static electricity to the film while unwrapping it for developing will appear as lightning on the processed film.

88. The glass wall and insulating oil acts as what type of filtration for X-ray photons generated in the tubehead?

   B. Inherent. Inherent filtration corresponds to the materials that X-ray photons encounter as they travel from the focal spot on the target to form the useful beam, primary radiation, outside the tube enclosure.

89. The total amount of radiation a dental patient receives

   D. is cumulative over a lifetime. The amount of radiation received is cumulative over the entire body. There are multiple sources, including radiation from the environment; however, the cumulative effect is the most significant issue.

90. Which tooth is missing?

   D. Number 30. Tooth number 30 (permanent mandibular first molar) is missing.

91. The radiolucent area involving the molar and premolars shows

   B. severe bone loss. The radiolucent area, particularly around teeth number 29 and number 31, shows severe bone loss typically associated with advanced periodontal disease.

92. Which of the following is one of the earliest clinical signs of overexposure to X-rays?

   B. Erythema. The earliest clinical sign of overexposure to X-rays is reddening (erythema) of the skin, also referred to as X-ray dermatitis.

93. Which of the following is considered to be the yearly maximum permissible dose (MPD) for dental patients?

   c. 10 mSv/0.1 REM. The annual MPD for the general public, including dental patients, is 10 mSv (0.1 REM) per year. This is one-tenth the dose permitted for dental personnel.

94. The primary purpose of monitoring X-ray equipment is to

   B. check for radiation leaks. X-ray equipment must be consistently monitored for leaking radiation that could harm unprotected staff and patients.

95. The primary advantage of an automatic film processor is that

   D. there is no need for chemicals. Automatic processors make developing films much easier than using a wet or manual process. Chemicals are still needed in order to produce an image.

96. During X-ray exposure, a thyroid collar should be placed on

   D. all patients. A thyroid collar, as well as a lead apron, must be used on all patients during X-ray exposure.

97. Radiation that has been deflected from its path by impact with matter is called

A. scatter radiation. Scatter radiation consists of rays from the primary beam that have deflected during their passage through tissues or other substances.

98. Leaving the radiograph in the final water bath too long will cause the image to

B. become clear. Radiographs should not be left in the water bath for more than 20 minutes or the emulsion will wash off and the film will become clear.

99. This radiograph is an example of a

A. bitewing radiograph. This radiograph is a bitewing radiograph, also referred to as an interproximal radiograph. The radiographic images of the coronal and cervical portions of both the maxillary and mandibular teeth and the alveolar borders of the given area are all recorded on this one film.

100. This radiograph illustrates the

B. left premolar. This radiograph is upside down. It is a left premolar bitewing radiograph. A premolar film should be positioned so that the exposure includes the distal aspect of the canine(s).

ANSWERS AND RATIONALES:
Infection Control (ICE)

1. Vaccination of employees against the hepatitis B virus must be offered within how many days following the start date of employment?

   C. 10 days. According to the OSHA Bloodborne Pathogen Standard, employees must be offered the hepatitis B vaccination series within 10 days following the start date of employment.

2. The MOST effective method of preventing cross-contamination in the dental office is

   D. performing proper handwashing. Handwashing is an excellent prevention method for indirect transmission, because infectious agents are often transmitted on objects that are physically handled.

3. Which of the following will determine that instrument sterilization was achieved?

   C. Biological monitors. Chemical indicators, physical monitors, and process integrators will identify which instruments have been processed, but they will not determine if sterilization was achieved.

4. A high-level disinfectant must have the ability to kill

   C. tuberculosis. High-level disinfectants are defined as a disinfectant that kills most, but not all, of *M. tuberculosis* spores.

5. Which of the following types of latex allergy is the MOST common?

   D. Irritant contact dermatitis. The most common type of latex allergy is irritant dermatitis, Type IV allergy. One sign of irritant dermatitis is a rash that is limited to the area of contact. Type I latex allergy is the most serious and can be life threatening.

6. Biofilm is made up of a thin film of

   A. colonized bacterial cells. Biofilm is a film of a dense, transparent, nonmineralized, highly organized colony of bacteria in a gel-like matrix

7. Dental instruments that are used in the mouth but do not penetrate tissue or bone are

   B. semicritical instruments. Semicritical instruments are used in the mouth and touch mucous membranes, but do not penetrate soft tissue or bone. Examples include the mouth mirror, impression trays, and amalgam condenser.

8. Who is responsible for supplying Material Safety Data Sheets to the dental office?

   C. Manufacturer. It is the manufacturer's responsibility to supply offices with an MSDS sheet; however, sheets may be obtained from the manufacturer, the distributor, or an available Internet site.

9. Coming into contact with which of the following is MOST likely to cause the spread of herpes in the dental office?

   D. Lesions. During the active infection, vesicles erupt that contain the herpes virus, which may be spread to others by direct contact with these lesions. For example, herpes can be spread from the lip lesion of one patient to the mouths of other dental patients via ungloved hands of a hygienist.

10. The main disadvantage to using a dry heat sterilizer is the

    C. long cycle time. A dry heat sterilizer requires a cycle time of 60–120 minutes. By contrast, a steam autoclave requires a cycle time of 15–30 minutes and a chemical vapor sterilizer requires a cycle time of 20 minutes.

11. The effects of chronic chemical toxicity include

    B. cancer. Chronic chemical toxicity involves being exposed to small amounts of chemicals over a long period of time. Effects of this type of exposure include cancer.

12. Critical items must be treated with which of the following methods to prevent the spread of infection?

    C. Sterilization. Critical items are items that penetrate skin and mucosa and must be disposed or sterilized to prevent cross-contamination.

13. Saliva ejectors and plastic high-volume evacuator tips should be

    A. disposed of after use. Plastic saliva ejectors and high-volume evacuator tips are considered to be expendables/disposable for single use only and are to be discarded.

14. An example of an engineering control is

    C. isolating or removing a hazard. An engineering control would include isolating or removing a hazard in order to decrease the chance of occupational exposure, such as using a puncture-resistant sharps container.

15. An example of a bloodborne pathogen is

    B. hepatitis C. Hepatitis A is transmitted through contaminated food and water. Tuberculosis and influenza are airborne pathogens. Hepatitis C is transmitted through blood and body fluids.

16. A positive biological monitoring test result indicates

    B. sterilization failed. Sterilization may have failed because of equipment malfunctions or operator error.

17. Which of the following is considered regulated waste?

    C. Used anesthetic needles. Used anesthetic needles must be disposed of in a leak-proof sharps container with a lid. Once the sharps container is filled, it must be disposed of properly through the use of a sharps waste contractor.

Infection Control

18. Which of the following agencies has the authority to enforce infection-control regulations?

D. Occupational Safety and Health Administration (OSHA). OSHA can enforce regulations. The CDC, ADA, and NIOSH can only make recommendations.

19. Destruction of all microorganisms is called

B. sterilization. Sterilization destroys all microorganisms, including viruses and bacterial spores, which are the most difficult to kill.

20. A chemical labeled a disinfectant is unable to kill

D. bacterial endospores. Disinfectants are unable to kill bacterial endospores. Only sterilants have the ability to kill bacterial endospores.

21. According to the OSHA Bloodborne Pathogen Standard, which of the following is prohibited in the dental operatory and sterilization areas?

C. Eating and drinking. Eating or drinking in the sterilization area is prohibited. Carpeting on the floor and cloth upholstery on chairs and stools should be avoided because they may harbor pathogens and are difficult to clean and disinfect. Study models do not need to be sterile because they are not placed in the oral cavity.

22. The safety and effectiveness of sterilization equipment in the dental office is controlled by the

D. Food and Drug Administration. The Food and Drug Administration is the federal agency that is responsible for overseeing the manufacturing, safety, and effectiveness of sterilization equipment.

23. Microorganisms that produce disease in humans are known as

B. pathogens. Pathogens are any virus, microorganism, or other substance that causes disease.

24. Which of the following tasks would require the dental assisting to wear utility gloves?

A. Disinfecting the operatory following patient care. Utility gloves will eliminate contact with chemicals during disinfection.

25. Which intermediate level disinfectant may contribute to staining of clinical surfaces?

B. Iodophors. Iodophors may contribute to staining clinical surfaces due to the iodine found in the solutions.

26. The agency dedicated to providing educational material to dental health professionals is the

C. OSAP. The Organization for Safety and Asepsis Procedures (OSAP) provides educational materials. The ADA is the national professional organization for dentists. The CDC and OSHA are involved with the safety and health of people and workers.

27. The patient notes on her medical history that she has active tuberculosis. She is scheduled for a crown preparation. How does her condition affect her dental treatment?

   C. Her treatment should be postponed until her disease is no longer active. Standard precautions do not protect the dental healthcare worker against transmission of tuberculosis, so no dental treatment should take place until the disease is no longer in an active phase.

28. To properly dispose of a blood-soaked gauze square, place it in

   A. a regulated trash bag. A blood-soaked gauze square is regulated medical waste and must be disposed of in a biohazard or regulated trash bag.

29. OSHA requires, which of the following dental employees receive training in the Bloodborne Pathogen Standard?

   C. Chairside assistant. OSHA requires that any employee with a reasonable risk of exposure to blood and body fluids should receive training in the Bloodborne Pathogen Standard both upon hire and annually.

30. Overgloves should be used when

   D. opening a drawer during patient treatment. Overgloves will prevent cross-contamination between contaminated exam gloves and the contents of the drawer.

31. The major advantage to using liquid chemical sterilization is that

   C. items that would be damaged by heat can be sterilized using this method. The disadvantages to this type of sterilization technique are the long exposure time required, which can range from 6–10 hours, and the effectiveness of sterilization cannot be verified

32. Which of the following conditions would contraindicate the use of nitrous oxide-oxygen conscious sedation?

   C. Nasal obstruction. To achieve the desired effect, nitrous oxide must be breathed deeply into the lungs. If the patient is unable to breathe deeply through their nose, the nitrous oxide will not be effective.

33. Sodium hypochlorite is recommended as a disinfectant for

   B. housekeeping surfaces. Because sodium hypochlorite is not an EPA-registered disinfectant, it is no longer recommended as an intermediate disinfectant for clinical contact areas.

34. Which of the following items should be disinfected before handling in the dental laboratory?

   C. Impression. Impressions are contaminated with saliva and other oral fluids and should always be disinfected before handling.

35. Which method of sterilization is recommended for items that will be used immediately after removal from the sterilizer?

   C. Flash sterilization. Items that will be used immediately after removal do not need to be bagged; therefore, they require a shorter sterilization time.

Infection Control

36. What type of water does the ADA and the CDC recommend when performing surgical procedures?

   B. Sterile water. To avoid postoperative infections, it is important to maintain sterility of instruments and materials, including the water used to irrigate the surgical wound.

37. What type of immunity occurs when a person receives a vaccination for a disease?

   B. Active artificial immunity. Active artificial immunity can also be called artificial acquired immunity.

38. Which mode of transmission involves contact with a contaminated instrument or surface?

   D. Indirect contact. Indirect contact occurs when the infectious agent is transferred to a second surface and then transmitted from there to a new host.

39. Microorganisms that accumulate on wet surfaces, such as on the inside of dental waterline tubing, are called

   B. biofilm. Biofilm is of concern in the dental profession because it may contain a variety of disease-causing pathogens.

40. Which of the following diseases is considered a chronic infection?

   C. Hepatitis B carrier state. A chronic disease is one that persists over a long period of time. It often stays in the body and periodically recurs.

41. Which of the following agencies would be LEAST concerned with infection control standards?

   B. FDA. The Food and Drug Administration (FDA) regulates manufacturing and labeling of medication and medical devices.

42. The MOST effective method of confirming sterilization of instruments is with

   C. bacterial spore testing. Bacterial spore testing is most effective for confirming sterilization. Chemical indicators, chemical integrators, and physical monitoring only indicate that an item was exposed to heat.

43. OSHA's Hazardous Communication Standard is concerned with preventing occupational exposure to dangerous

   B. chemicals. This standard is designed to protect the worker from exposure to dangerous chemicals and materials.

44. Which of the following conditions could cause poor healing after oral surgery?

   B. Poorly controlled diabetes. Poorly controlled diabetes reduces the body's ability to fight infection and can lead to poor healing after surgery.

45. The best way to ensure immunity is by

   A. vaccination. Vaccines consist of tiny amounts of the antigen, which stimulate the body to produce antibodies.

46. Which of the following diseases is easily transmitted in the healthcare setting?

    C. MRSA. MRSA, or methicillin-resistant *Staphylococcus aureus*, is a strain of bacteria that is resistant to traditional antibiotics and is a common infection transmitted in the healthcare setting. HIV/AIDS and tuberculosis usually require prolonged exposure to the pathogen, and hepatitis A is transmitted through contaminated food and water.

47. What is the mechanism of action of the autoclave sterilizer?

    B. Steam under pressure. Sterilization by the autoclave occurs when steam reaches high pressure, destroying the pathogens.

48. The first handwashing of each day should include a

    B. soft brush to scrub nails. At the beginning of each day, clinical staff members should wash thoroughly including the use of a soft scrub brush to clean around fingernails.

49. Extracted teeth are

    B. regulated waste. Extracted teeth are regulated waste and must be disposed of properly in a biohazard container. Extracted teeth without amalgam restorations can be placed in the sterilizer prior to disposal.

50. According to OSHA, the Hepatitis B vaccine is to be made available to employees at risk for contamination. The employee is responsible for

    C. arriving on time for the appointment. According to OSHA standards, the employer is responsible for all costs associated with the immunization process. It is the staff member's obligation to show up on time for the immunization appointment.

51. Which of the following procedures is relevant to OSHA's Bloodborne Pathogen Standard?

    C. Hepatitis B immunization. Immunizations for Hepatitis B are required as part of OSHA's Bloodborne Pathogen Standard to protect the worker against communicable diseases.

52. Approximately how much of the waste generated in the dental office is hazardous?

    A. 3%. Infectious waste in the dental office is a small portion of the total waste: approximately 3%.

53. The main disadvantage of using a dry heat sterilizer is the

    A. damage to heat-sensitive items. The very high heat of the dry heat sterilizer can melt or damage some items like plastics and paper. Dry heat does not corrode metal, and both closed containers and live spore testing may be used with this method of sterilization.

54. Gauze that has had contact with bodily fluids, such as blood and/or saliva, is what type of waste?

    C. Infectious. Infectious waste is any waste that has the ability to transmit disease. This is also known as regulated waste.

55. Which of the following PPE (personal protective equipment) is used to prevent inhalation of droplets and/or spatter?

    C. Mask. Masks cover the nose and mouth to prevent inhalation of droplets and/or spatter.

Infection Control

56. What is the purpose of a barrier in infection control?

> **B. Disrupt the transfer of infectious agents.** The purpose of infection control is to erect barriers that cause disruptions in the transfer of infectious agents.

57. Used barriers and paper from the dental office are classified as what type of waste?

> **B. Nonregulated.** Most of the waste produced by the dental office is considered nonregulated waste. Only those items that are saturated with blood or body fluids or that are from living tissue are considered regulated waste.

58. Bacteria that must have oxygen to grow and live are considered

> **B. aerobic bacteria.** Aerobic bacteria need oxygen. Anaerobic bacteria do not require oxygen to grow and live.

59. When bacteria form a protective coat of protein around themselves, they are known as

> **C. spores.** In order to defend themselves from destruction, some bacteria will form a dense, thick wall of protein, making them extremely resistant to heat, drying, and chemicals. In this form, they are known as spores or endospores.

60. Which of the following may be used as a surface disinfectant in the dental office?

> **A. Iodophors.** Iodophors and synthetic phenol compounds are accepted for surface disinfection. Ethyl alcohol and isopropyl alcohol are not effective in the presence of bioburden such as blood and saliva. The ADA, CDC, and OSAP do not recommend alcohol as an environmental surface disinfectant.

61. Routine handwashing will remove

> **B. transient microflora.** The resident microflora are the normal microbial inhabitants of the skin and are not considered to be harmful. Transient microflora are the microbes picked up by touching surfaces and are not only most likely to cause disease but they are easily removed by thorough handwashing.

62. Which of the following is a pathogenic waste?

> **C. Extracted teeth.** Teeth and other waste tissues are infectious pathogenic waste and must be disposed of in a leak-proof container or biohazard bag.

63. Any reusable item intended for patient care should be

> **D. heat sterilized after use.** Covering a reusable item will not prevent contamination. All instruments that are not heat sensitive must be processed in a sterilizer. Heat-sensitive items must be soaked in a liquid sterilant for the time recommended by the manufacturer.

64. Of the following choices, which one would reflect the purpose of OSHA Standards MOST accurately?

> **A. It is the law and enforceable.** Regulations are laws that must be followed. They are issued by governmental entities, such as OSHA.

65. The primary advantage of using disposable items in a dental office is

> **B. reduced cross-contamination.** The primary advantage of using disposables is the prevention of cross-contamination. Unfortunately, most are made of nonbiodegradable plastics and are not eco-friendly.

66. Which of the following chemicals can be used as an immersion disinfectant/sterilant for instruments?

> **B. Glutaraldehyde.** Glutaraldehydes are high-level disinfectants/sterilants designed for immersion for long periods (6–10 hours). Iodophors, sodium hypochlorite, and synthetic phenols are intermediate level surface disinfectants and are not intended for immersion.

67. What is the appropriate PPE when processing instruments in the ultrasonic cleaner?

> **C. Utility gloves, mask, safety glasses, and gown.** Processing contaminated instruments in the ultrasonic bath carries a strong risk of accidental puncture for the dental assistant. Use of heavy-duty utility gloves, as well as full PPE, offers more protection than examination, food handler, or double examination gloves.

68. An infection with a short duration is called

> **C. acute.** An acute infection is one that has a rapid onset and/or a short course.

69. A needlestick injury could transmit disease. This type of disease transmission is called

> **B. parenteral.** Parenteral transmission is through the skin, such as with a needlestick. Enteral transmission is transmission through the gastrointestinal track. An opportunistic infection takes advantage of the weakened immune status of the patient to cause disease, and a vector-borne transmission usually involves an insect.

70. After treatment, using a low-level disinfectant-type cleaner on the bagged dental chair

> **C. provides additional asepsis.** Using a bag to cover the dental chair during treatment will assist in reducing the bioburden on the chair; however, once the bag is removed, the chair should be sprayed with a low-level disinfectant to begin killing existing microbes.

71. Which of the following actions is MOST appropriate during an OSHA inspection?

> **C. Compliance with inspector, without volunteering information.** The office must comply with all requests made by the inspector; however, unless specifically requested, do not offer any information that is not directly asked for.

72. Which of the following is the best choice for cleaning the dental vacuum system?

> **A. Nonfoaming, enzymatic cleaner.** The suction system in a dental office is contaminated with protein residues from blood and saliva that can be broken down by the enzymatic component of the cleaner. Foaming agents could clog the lines and should be avoided. Bleach can damage the metal components of the unit.

73. Prior to placing instruments into a sterilizer, they must be precleaned in a/an

> **C. ultrasonic unit.** The first step in the sterilization procedure is to preclean the instruments, which typically includes ultrasonic cleaning. An FDA instrument dishwasher may also be used.

Infection Control

74. Which of the following organizations is the authority for infection control education?

C. Organization for Safety and Asepsis Procedures. OSAP is listed as dentistry's authority for infection control information.

75. Which of the following is the MOST effective mouth rinse to use prior to a dental appointment?

B. Chlorhexidine. Chlorhexidine mouth rinse is a long-lasting, antimicrobial mouth rinse that can reduce the level of oral microorganisms for up to 5 hours. This is especially important for procedures where a rubber dam will not be used.

76. Which of the following is the LEAST likely route to a hazardous chemical exposure?

B. Mucous membrane splash. The most common routes to chemical exposure are direct contact with the skin and accidently or deliberately ingesting and breathing in vapors.

77. Which of the following surface disinfectants is tuberculocidal?

A. Iodophor. Iodophors are approved as intermediate-level surface disinfectants that include tuberculocidal action. Glutaraldehyde is not a surface disinfectant, and neither bleach nor quaternary ammonias are accepted as tuberculocidal agents.

78. Which surface is likely to become contaminated in a dental operatory during a procedure?

B. Clinical contact surfaces. The surfaces most likely to be contaminated during patient care include the headrest, chair controls, counter tops, light handles, handpieces, hoses, and other items touched by gloved hands or aerosol from the procedure.

79. Which of the following is a noncritical instrument?

D. X-ray tubehead. The x-ray tubehead is a noncritical instrument because it does not go into the oral cavity and only touches intact skin.

80. An example of a percutaneous injury is

B. a needlestick from a sharps container. A needlestick is a percutaneous injury. Percutaneous means "through the skin."

81. If mercury is spilled in the office, it should be cleaned up using a/an

C. spill kit. Every office that uses amalgam should have an emergency spill kit. The individual cleaning up the spill should wear PPE and not handle the material with bare hands or use a vacuum cleaner to pick up the spill.

82. Which of the following items produces the most aerosol and splatter?

B. High-speed handpiece. The combination of water spray with the high-speed rotations of the handpiece spreads large amounts of splatter and aerosols into the air around the treatment zone.

Infection Control

83. Scrap amalgam should be

  B. stored in an airtight container. Mercury is a toxic metal that, when mixed with dental alloy, must be disposed of aseptically. Amalgam containing mercury should be stored in an airtight container under water or in a special chemically treated receptacle.

84. *Legionella* bacteria can cause what type of infection in humans?

  D. Pneumonia. *Legionella* bacteria are transmitted by inhalation of aerosolized contaminated water, which causes pneumonia.

85. The purpose of the ultrasonic cleaner is to

  B. remove debris from instruments prior to sterilization. The ultrasonic cleaner removes debris or bioburden from instruments so sterilization can be effective. It is a cleaning step, but not a disinfecting or sterilization step.

86. Instruments used on amalgam restorations should be cleaned of all debris prior to autoclaving because amalgam

  A. releases free vapor when heated. Because the heating of amalgam can cause free vapor, operatories and sterilization areas should be well ventilated. All residual amalgam should be removed from the instruments and stored aseptically.

87. The last PPE put on before beginning patient treatment must be the

  C. gloves. Gloves are put on last in order to avoid contaminating them before they are used in the patient's mouth.

88. Nitrous oxide exposure in the dental office can be reduced by

  C. using a scavenger system. A scavenger system reduces the N_2O that escapes and is inhaled.

89. Who is MOST likely to be a susceptible host to pathogenic agents?

  C. Person with HIV. A person with a weakened immune system does not have the resistance to fight off the chance of infection and becomes a susceptible host. This is especially true if the causative agent is present in large quantities and is highly virulent.

90. The main goal of an effective infection control plan in a dental office is to

  A. reduce the number of microbes. Effective infection control reduces the number of microbes in the office by the use of barriers, PPE, disposable items, and adequate disinfection and sterilization techniques.

91. Items that cannot be placed in the autoclave but are reusable are classified as

  B. semicritical items. Whenever possible, items that cannot be heat sterilized should be disposed of. An instrument that can be harmed by heat should be placed in a liquid sterilization solution for 6 to 10 hours.

Infection Control

Infection Control

92. Orthodontic bands and wires, burs, scalpel blades, and suture needles are

   A. sharps. Sharps items include orthodontic bands and wires, dental burs, scalpel blades, suture needles, as well as injection and suture needles, broken instruments, and glass. Sharps are treated and disposed of as infectious waste.

93. Potable water is another name for

   B. drinking water. Potable or drinking water is monitored using standards set by the Environmental Protection Agency.

94. Which of the following is a required safety measure when using a curing light?

   C. Tinted safety glasses. The visible light spectrum of the curing light is damaging to the eyes. Tinted safety lenses or a shield on the unit should be used to protect both staff and patient.

95. To be effective, surface barriers should be

   B. fluid resistant. To be effective, surface barriers need to be resistant to fluids. Fluid-resistant barriers prevent microorganisms in blood, saliva, and liquids from soaking through the barrier material and contacting the underlying surface.

96. Patients who close their lips around the saliva ejector to clear their mouths run the risk of what type of contamination?

   C. Patient to patient. Research has shown that if a patient closes their mouth around the saliva ejector, there can be a reverse flow in the vacuum line.

97. The MOST resistant form of known life is a/an

   C. spore. Spores can survive extremes of heat and dryness and even the presence of disinfectants and radiation.

98. How would a dental assistant ensure that cross-contamination does not occur when a patient's denture is polished in the lab?

   C. Use only disposable or sterilized polishing materials. Laboratory items such as burs and handpieces should be sterilized between patients. Pumice and rag wheels should either be disposed of or sterilized after use.

99. How often should a face mask be replaced?

   A. Between patients. Because the outer surface of the face mask becomes contaminated during dental procedures with droplets created by sprays from patient fluids and dental handpieces, the face mask should always be changed between patients and during patient treatment if the mask becomes wet.

100. The name of the cleaning technique used at the end of a patient appointment is the

   A. spray-wipe-spray. Spray-wipe-spray technique recommends that, at the end of patient care, bags should be removed and discarded, the unit be sprayed with a surface disinfectant and wiped down vigorously, then sprayed and allowed to stay wet for 10 minutes. After 10 minutes, wipe away any remaining disinfectant and rebag the unit.

NOTES

NOTES

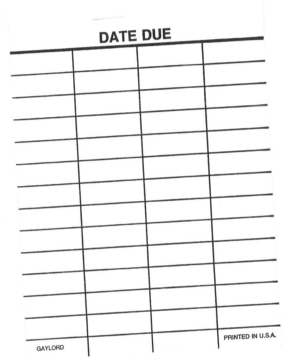

RRS1102